Topics in Neuroscience

Managing Editor:

GIANCARLO COMI

Co-Editor:

JACOPO MELDOLESI

Associate Editors:

UGO ECARI

MASSIMO FILIPPI

GIANVITO MARTINO

Springer

Milano
Berlin
Heidelberg
New York
Hong Kong
London
Paris
Tokyo

M. Filippi • G. Comi (Eds)

New Frontiers of MR-based Techniques in Multiple Sclerosis

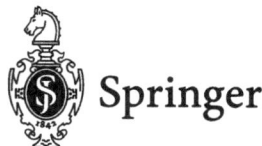 Springer

MASSIMO FILIPPI
Neuroimaging Research Unit
Department of Neuroscience
Scientific Institute and University
Ospedale San Raffaele, Milan, Italy

GIANCARLO COMI
Department of Neurology
Scientific Institute and University
Ospedale San Raffaele, Milan, Italy

The Editors and Authors wish to thank SCHERING S.p.A. for the support and help in the realization and promotion of this volume

Springer-Verlag Italia
a member of BertelsmannSpringer Science+Business Media GmbH

© Springer-Verlag Italia, Milano 2003
Softcover reprint of the hardcover 1st edition 2003

http://www.springer.de

ISBN-13: 978-88-470-2239-3   e-ISBN-13: 978-88-470-2237-9
DOI: 10.1007/978-88-470-2237-9

Library of Congress Cataloging-in-Publication Data:
New fronteers [i.e. frontiers] of MR-based techniques in multiple sclerosis / M. Filippi, G. Comi, eds.
p. ; cm. -- (Topics in neuroscience)
"The result of an international workshop held in Milan on June 1st, 2002 during the
Sixth Annual Advanced Course on the Use of Magnetic Resonance Techniques in
Multiple Sclerosis" - Introd.
Include bibliographical references and index.
ISBN-13: 978-88-470-2239-3
1. Multiple sclerosis--Magnetic resonance imaging--Congresses. I. Title: New frontiers
of MR-based techniques in multiple sclerosis. II. Filippi M. (Massimo), 1961 - III. Comi,
G. (Giancarlo), 1947 - IV. Advanced Course on the Use of Magnetic Resonance
Techniques in Multiple Sclerosis (6th : 2002 : Milan, Italy) V. Series.
[DNLM: 1. Multiple Sclerosis--diagnosis. 2. Magnetic Resonance Imaging--methods.
3. Magnetic Resonance Spectroscopy--methods. WL 360 N532 2003]
RC377 .N49 2003
616.8'3407548--dc21

2002191123

Typesetting: Copy Card Center s.r.l. (Milan)

Cover design: Simona Colombo

SPIN: 10900895

Foreword

Magnetic resonance in multiple sclerosis has been a fascinating topic for study over the last 15 years. The changes that occur on proton density and T2-weighted imaging have been measured in a number of natural history studies and in clinical trials. More recently gadolinium enhancement, as a sign of activity, and the measurement of hypointensity on T1-weighted imaging related to both acute and chronic black holes have been measured. The correlations between clinical measures and MRI measures have been positive but modest. MRI measures are probably stronger as a predictor for the future then they are for an assessment of how the patient is doing at the present moment. The most precise correlation of magnetic resonance is with the chronic pathology. The correlation between MRI and the acute inflammatory pathology is much less consistent: a great deal of additional data needs to be collected in this regard.

However, as a measure of chronic pathology, MRI is quite precise. Therefore, MRI measures of activity and MRI measures of the extent of disease have been shown to be important and sensitive measures of both disease activity and treatment effects.

Newer MR techniques have now the potential to be pathologically much more specific. For example, conventional MRI measures have shown us the following:

1. The extent of disease on proton density is very sensitive to changes seen over time and for treatment effects. There is a dynamic of the disease that is apparent on MRI that is not seen clinically; in fact, activity may be almost continuous in some patients. The changes on proton density imaging are pathologically nonspecific, but distinctions can be deducted from the use of frequent and systematic scans over time, allowing some retrospective insight into the differentiation of inflammatory versus chronic pathology.

2. T1 hypointensities (black holes) can develop as an acute dynamic change similar to that seen on proton density or as a chronic change with pathological features related to destructive elements of pathology such as axonal loss and gliosis.

3. Gadolinium enhancement is a very good measure of blood brain barrier disruption and of the degree and extent of inflammation in acutely active lesions.

More recently, such techniques as MR spectroscopy can reveal local and global changes that reflect axonal damage and, if sustained, axonal loss.

In this volume, spectroscopy and other techniques such as magnetization transfer imaging, diffusion imaging, perfusion imaging, and functional MRI are discussed with regard to how they have been or can be applied to the understanding of the evolution of brain pathology in multiple sclerosis.

High field imaging is now available at three tesla (3T) up to eight tesla (8T). The final chapter in this book discusses the advantages and the problems related to high field imaging.

The Holy Grail of systematic MRI in MS is to estimate and eventually measure the evolution of the pathology both in respect of individual lesions and in respect of the total extent of disease. There is even some tantalizing evidence that magnetic resonance spectroscopy, early in the disease, may identify patients with poor prognosis. Data now exist to suggest that the number of MRI lesions seen early on the proton density scan are important in predicting a poor prognosis. Therefore, combinations of these MR measures, properly understood, could help us to select out patients for aggressive therapy based on their long-term prognosis.

In order to make decisions on a rational basis, however, we must have prospective information from cohorts of patients studied from early and followed for long periods of time.

I invite you to enjoy these review articles that help to explain the various MR techniques and how they can be applied to understanding MS.

Donald W. Paty, MD, FRCPC
Professor Emeritus
The University of British Columbia
Vancouver Hospital
Vancouver, Canada

Table of Contents

List of Contributors

E.C. Bourekas
Department of Radiology,
The Ohio State University, Columbus,
Ohio, USA
e-mail: bourekas.1@osu.edu

B. Brochet
Laboratory of Neurobiology of Myelin
Disorders, University Victor Segalen
Bordeaux 2, Bordeaux, France
e-mail: bruno.brochet@chu-bordeaux.fr

J.-M. Caille
Laboratory of Neurobiology of Myelin
Disorders, University Victor Segalen
Bordeaux 2, Bordeaux, France
e-mail: jean-marie.caille@chu-bordeaux.fr

D.W. Chakeres
Department of Radiology
The Ohio State University, Columbus,
Ohio, USA
e-mail: chakeres.1@osu.edu

G. Comi
Department of Neurology,
Scientific Institute and University
Ospedale San Raffaele, Milan, Italy
e-mail: g.comi@hrs.it

V. Dousset
Laboratory of Neurobiology of Myelin
Disorders, University Victor Segalen
Bordeaux 2, Bordeaux, France
e-mail: vincent.dousset@chu-bordeaux.fr

M. Filippi
Neuroimaging Research Unit,
Department of Neuroscience, Scientific
Institute and University Ospedale
San Raffaele, Milan, Italy
e-mail: filippi.massimo@hsr.it

O. Gonen
Department of Radiology,
New York University School of Medicine,
New York, USA
e-mail: oded.gonen@med.nyu.edu

R.I. Grossman
Department of Radiology,
New York University School of Medicine,
New York, USA
e-mail: robert.grossman@med.nyu.edu

A. Kangarlu
Department of Radiology,
The Ohio State University,
Columbus, Ohio, USA
e-mail: kangarlu@justice.med.ohio-state.edu

D.H. Miller
Department of Neuroinflammation,
NMR Research Unit, Institute
of Neurology, London, UK
e-mail: d.miller@ion.ucl.ac.uk

K.G. Petry
Laboratory of Neurobiology of Myelin
Disorders, University Victor Segalen
Bordeaux 2, Bordeaux, France
e-mail: klaus.petry@bordeaux.inserm.fr

K.W. Rammohan
Department of Neurology,
The Ohio State University,
Columbus, Ohio, USA
e-mail: rammohan.2 @osu.edu

W. Rashid
Department of Neuroinflammation,
NMR Research Unit,
Institute of Neurology, London, UK
e-mail: w.rashid@ion.ucl.ac.uk

M. Rovaris
Neuroimaging Research Unit,
Department of Neuroscience,
Scientific Institute and University
Ospedale San Raffaele, Milan, Italy
e-mail: rovaris.marco@hsr.it

M.A. Rocca
Neuroimaging Research Unit,
Departement of Neuroscience, Scientific
Institute and University Ospedale San
Raffaele, Milan, Italy
e-mail: mara.rocca@hsr.it

Introduction

M. FILIPPI, M. ROVARIS, G. COMI

There is no doubt that the application of conventional magnetic resonance imaging (MRI) to the study of multiple sclerosis (MS) has greatly improved our ability to diagnose this condition and to monitor its evolution. The exquisite sensitivity of T2-weighted MRI in the detection of MS lesions, together with the ability of postcontrast T1-weighted images to reflect the presence of increased blood-brain barrier (BBB) permeability associated with inflammatory activity, allow us to demonstrate the spatial and temporal dissemination of MS lesions earlier than is possible from a clinical assessment of the patients. In addition, serial MRI scanning of the brain is five to ten times more sensitive for detecting disease activity than the clinical evaluation of relapses. In consequence, metrics derived from conventional MRI are now established, in conjunction with the clinical assessment, as outcome measures by which to monitor the efficacy of experimental treatments in placebo-controlled MS trials.

Nevertheless, although conventional MRI has improved our understanding of how MS evolves, the information it provides about the disease pathology is limited in both accuracy and specificity. T2-weighted signal abnormalities reflect just the presence of increased water content, independent of the severity of the associated tissue disruption, which may range from transient edema to irreversible demyelination and axonal loss. The presence of contrast enhancement indicates that BBB is locally disrupted, but it says nothing about the extent and severity of the inflammatory phase, the constitution of its cellular components, or the resultant tissue damage. In addition, conventional MRI is unable to detect and quantify the presence of MS-related damage occurring in the so-called normal-appearing tissues. These limitations of the technique can at least partially explain the modest correlation observed in many studies between conventional MRI findings and MS patients' clinical status. As a consequence, in the past few years there have been impressive advances in the implementation of modern MRI techniques for the assessment of MS patients, with the ultimate goal of defining reliable MRI markers of MS evolution. There is now general agreement that these markers must be quantitative, in order to grade precisely the extent of tissue damage; they should provide information about the most destructive aspects of the disease, the leading factors in causing MS irreversible disability; and they must enable study of (at least) the entire brain, since MS is a widespread disease affecting all the tissues of the central nervous system (CNS). The definition of reliable MRI markers is particularly urgent now that there is partially effective treatment for MS, and the ability to conduct large placebo-controlled trials is therefore limited.

Structural and metabolic quantitative MRI techniques, such as magnetization transfer (MT) MRI, diffusion-weighted (DW) MRI, and proton MR spectroscopy (^{1}H-MRS), are increasingly being used to monitor MS evolution. Other modern MRI techniques, such as functional MRI (fMRI), cell-specific MRI, perfusion MRI, and microscopic imaging with ultra-high-field MR scanners, are emerging as additional promising tools for improving our understanding of the pathophysiology of MS. These various MRI techniques represent an extraordinary set of powerful instruments by which to gain in vivo fundamental insights into the disease process.

MT and DW MRI enable us to quantify the extent of structural changes occurring in T2-visible lesions and in tissue that appears normal on conventional MRI. Both these techniques have the ability to provide quantitative and continuous measures. While MT MRI-derived metrics seem to reflect predominantly demyelination and loss of axons, the pathological substrates of DW MRI changes are less clearly defined. Nevertheless, measures derived from DW MRI can give in vivo information about the size, shape, geometry, and orientation of tissues, which look promising for a more accurate depiction of MS-related white matter tract disruption. Both MT and DW MRI are able to provide information about MS injury to at least large portions of the brain, and their application to the study of specific CNS structures such as the spinal cord and optic nerves is being optimized. MT MRI quantities have been found to be reproducible and sensitive to MS changes over 1-3 years, whereas the reproducibility and sensitivity to disease changes of DW MRI-derived metrics are currently unknown. As a consequence, although they are possible, the optimization and standardization across multiple sites and over time of MT MRI and DW MRI can be challenging. In addition, for both these techniques, long-term longitudinal studies of MS patients are also warranted to better define the predictive value of observed changes for the subsequent evolution of the disease.

With respect to MT and DW MRI, ^{1}H-MRS can add information on the biochemical nature of MS-related changes, with the potential to improve significantly our ability to monitor inflammatory demyelination and axonal injury. Axonal damage and loss can be quantified through the measurement of N-acetylaspartate (NAA), a metabolite which in adult human brains is localized almost exclusively within neurons and neuronal processes. In MS patients, the NAA levels of T2-visible lesions and normal-appearing brain tissue correlate strongly with clinical disability, and NAA measurements are sensitive to disease changes over time. The feasibility of whole-brain NAA measurements is a major advancement in the field that has the potential to provide an overall and highly specific marker of MS severity. However, ^{1}H-MRS is time-consuming and technically demanding, and its optimization and standardization across multiple sites in the context of large-scale studies remains challenging.

There is increasing evidence that various mechanisms active during and after MS injury to the CNS have the potential to limit the functional consequences of the disease-related structural damage. These mechanisms are likely to contribute to the observed variability of the clinical disease severity in patients with similar MRI-measurable disease burdens. Some of these mechanisms, such as resolution of edema and inflammation and remyelination, can be monitored using the above-mentioned structural and metabolic MR techniques. fMRI, which enables us to detect brain areas where local blood flow is increased as a consequence of neuronal activity during task performance, holds substantial promise for elucidating the mechanisms of cortical adaptive reorganization following irreversible MS damage. The application of fMRI to the study of MS is limited by the need to select patients with a high degree of compliance and without severe deficits affecting the performance of specific tasks. In addition, the reproducibility of fMRI results is still unclear, and there is an urgent need to acquire longitudinal data for proper validation of the technique.

Cellular MRI and perfusion MRI have the potential to improve our ability to monitor the various aspects of MS inflammation. This would represent a major achievement in our understanding of the pathogenesis of new lesion formation and evolution. Preliminary cell-specific MRI studies with contrast media sensitive to the presence of macrophages have shown that there are a number of MS lesions where cell trafficking is likely to occur in the absence of gadolinium enhancement. Understanding the pathological heterogeneity of active MS lesions might be useful for better elucidation of the disease pathobiology.

Although the safety of field strengths above 3 T has not yet been established, high-field MRI will affect dramatically anatomical visualization, proton and nonproton MRS, fMRI, and nonproton imaging and thus our ability to image some of the critical components of the disease. This area of MR technology is moving rapidly, and the time for more extensive clinical application of high-field MRI will probably come soon.

The strengths and weaknesses of all these modern quantitative MRI techniques for the study of MS are extensively covered in this book, which is the result of an International Workshop held in Milan on 1 June 2002, during the Sixth Annual Advanced Course on the Use of Magnetic Resonance Techniques in Multiple Sclerosis. The book also provides a valuable summary of the state of the art, as well as defining areas for future research in the field.

Chapter 1

Cell-Specific Imaging in Pathologic Conditions of the Central Nervous System, with Special Reference to Multiple Sclerosis

V. DOUSSET, B. BROCHET, J.-M. CAILLE, K.G. PETRY

In vivo cell-specific imaging

Multiple Sclerosis and Experimental Autoimmune Encephalomyelitis

As in other autoimmune diseases, the inflammatory process of multiple sclerosis (MS) implicates T cells, B cells, and macrophages, and the activation of local organ-specific phagocytic cells. Particular to MS is the infiltration of the lymphocytes into the central nervous system (CNS) by crossing the blood-brain barrier (BBB) and the activation of the intrinsic immunoeffector microglia cells and of astrocytes. Although the pathologic lesions involving the brain and the spinal cord in MS can be visualized in vivo using both routine and more specific magnetic resonance imaging (MRI) techniques [1], the cellular events of CNS inflammation are difficult to observe in vivo.

Recent advances in both cell tracer technology and cell biology, however, have provided new tools for specific cell labeling that may in the future allow significant biomedical applications to be developed, mainly in the treatment of some neurodegenerative pathologies of the CNS or in demyelinating diseases such as MS. Most recent progress in specific cell labeling has been achieved by using the biological function of professional phagocytes, in particular cells of the mononuclear phagocytic system and the pharmacokinetic property of some MRI contrast agents of being captured by these cells.

Biocompatible dextran-coated iron oxide nanoparticles have been used with MRI for several years. Labeling of lymphocytes with these particles does not cause cytotoxicity or alterations in biodistribution or in normal physiologic lymphocyte functions such as cell adhesion to the vascular endothelium [2-4]. Superparamagnetic iron oxide (SPIO) has been used in liver imaging as macrophagic liver cells (Kupffer cells) rapidly phagocytose the SPIO after intravenous injection. The ultrasmall superparamagnetic iron oxide (USPIO), with a mean particle size of 20 nm (Sinerem, Laboratoire Guerbet, Aulnay, France, and Combidex, Advanced Magnetics, Cambridge, Mass., USA), evades the hepatic filter and accumulates preferentially in the macrophagic cells of other tissues, especially in the lymph nodes [5-8].

Professional phagocytes (macrophages of hematomonocytic origin and activated resident microglia) are involved in all steps of MS lesion development. Macrophages accompany the T lymphocytes during inflammation, they remove the myelin debris (lipid-laden macrophages), and they are present during the process of myelin repair [9]. Consequently, USPIO has been recently proposed for use in imaging the accumulation of macrophages in the brain suffering from MS [10-12]. In the acute experimental autoimmune encephalomyelitis (EAE) model of MS induced in Lewis rats, USPIO (AMI-227, Sinerem) was tested for its ability to show in vivo lesions associated with macrophage activity. In these studies, 24 h after intravenous injection of USPIO, EAE lesions associated with marked macrophage activity were seen on MRI as increased signal intensities in T1-weighted images and as low signal intensities in T2-weighted images (Fig. 1). Electron microscopy demonstrated the presence of iron particles within the cytoplasm of phagocytic cells and confirmed that the major uptake is either by activated microglia or by blood monocytes or both, which have actively transported

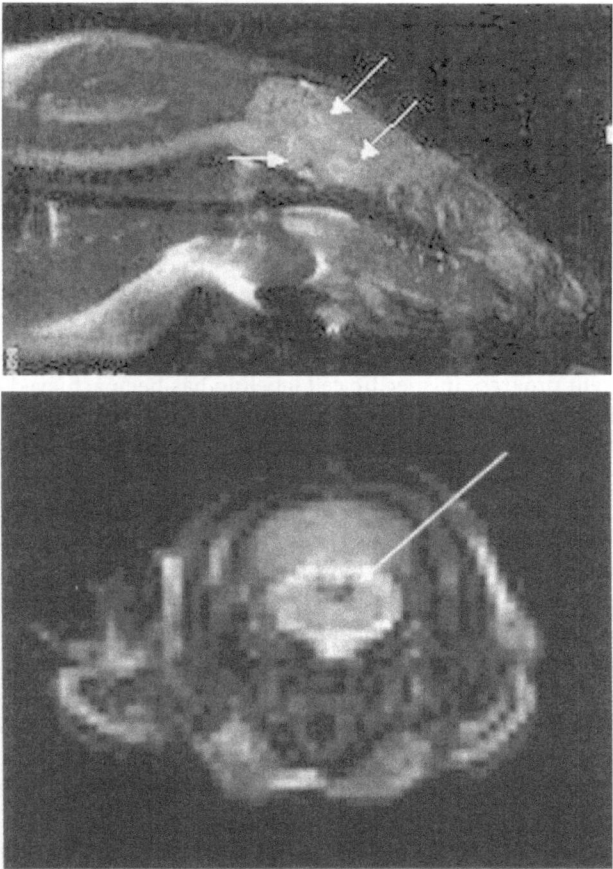

Fig. 1. Sagittal T1-weighted image (*top*) and coronal T2*-weighted image (*bottom*) of a rat brain with clinical EAE. *Arrows* indicate the lesion area

the USPIO to the site of inflammation through the BBB. These studies, performed in acute as well in remitting-relapsing rat EAE models of MS, confirm the capacity of MRI to show USPIO-labeled macrophages in inflammatory lesions of the CNS.

In relation to other MRI techniques using traditional contrast agents such as gadolinium that indicate passive breakdown of the BBB, important differences were observed. EAE lesions not enhanced by gadolinium can be seen after intravenous injection of USPIO [11], suggesting infiltration of macrophages into the brain parenchyma without or before rupture of the BBB.

Preliminary cell-specific imaging studies with USPIO in MS patients (phase IIa studies) have also revealed the presence of inflammatory brain lesions. During acute relapses three patterns of inflammation were observed using both gadolinium and USPIO: i) most of the lesions enhanced with both gadolinium and USPIO; ii) some of the lesions enhanced with gadolinium only and iii) some enhanced with USPIO only, suggesting that USPIO and gadolinium give different information about the nature of inflammatory lesions. USPIO used in vivo in MRI as a specific marker for macrophages within the CNS could reveal the cellular aspect of the inflammatory lesions in which macrophages are active, as opposed to gadolinium, which indicates passive breakdown of the BBB [13].

Another paramagnetic small-particle iron oxide agent, MION-46L, has been used in mouse EAE [14]. The agent was visualized by MRI performed 6 h after intraveous injection in lesions where it was localized by histopathologic study to the vascular endothelium, the perivascular space, and macrophages within perivascular cuffs and areas of inflammation and demyelination. Differences in these observations to specific macrophage labeling in EAE lesions suggest that the scanning delay is a critical parameter in cell-specific macrophage activity imaging with USPIO [12].

Ischemic Injury

As in inflammatory brain pathology, cells of the mononuclear phagocytotic system infiltrate ischemic tissue and can potentially aggravate tissue damage. Recent attempts have used USPIO cell labeling to visualize the demarcation of tissue believed to be affected from intact tissue, and to monitor macrophage activity after focal acute cerebral ischemia [15-17].

Tumor Delineation

Other CNS cells in pathophysiologic circumstances can be targeted by USPIO. Experimentally, tumor cells have revealed their capacity to capture USPIO given by intravenous injection. Imaging of glioma in humans may also be promising, first, because tumor cells may be revealed by their phagocytic activity and, secondly, because tumors are accompanied by macrophages [18, 19] or activated microglia, as shown in rat glioma [20]. Magnetic labeling of macrophages and microglia with USPIO provides prolonged and precise delineation of the margins of brain tumors. As microglia cells play a very sensitive and crucial role in the response to almost any brain pathology where they are activated to a phagocytic state, microglia labeling may further reflect the immunologic reaction of the CNS to glioma.

In Vitro Cell-Specific Labeling and In Vivo Tracking for Cell Therapy

Recent work on stem cells of the mammalian CNS, particularly in man, has indicated new hope for the treatment of many neurodegenerative diseases or CNS injuries [21] as these cells are able to proliferate and to differentiate into neurons, astrocytes, and oligodendrocytes. Their potential for plasticity is even greater than originally imagined. Transplanted into bone marrow of irradiated mice, they give rise to "normal" blood cells [22]. Conversely, stem cells from the bone marrow can differentiate into cells of the CNS such as microglia and astrocytes [23], and stromal bone marrow cells can develop a neuronal phenotype in vitro [24, 25] and can also migrate to the brain parenchyma after intravenous injection. These cells convey neuronal antigens and may differentiate into neurons in vivo [26, 27].

To promote cell intervention within the CNS, either stereotaxic implantation of cell preparations in the CNS or cell trafficking across the BBB is used. SPIO targeted to the transferrin receptor has been used for MRI monitoring of oligodendrocyte progenitors transplanted into the spinal cord of myelin-deficient rats [28]. Cells were incubated in vitro with the particles before transplantation. Migration of transplanted cells along the spinal cord was seen by MRI. This technique would be useful to monitor future transplantation-repairing strategies in MS and in other human dysmyelinating diseases, e.g., Pelizaeus-Merzbacher disease [29].

In vitro, CD34+ hematopoietic cells and equivalent Sca1+ rat cells isolated from bone marrow [30] and human peripheral blood lymphocytes and monocytes from MS patients can be labeled intracellularly with dextran-coated iron particles [31]. Twenty-four hours after intravenous injection into immunodeficient mice, USPIO-labeled CD34+ hematopoietic cells can be detected in several organs [32]. Magnetic labeling ex vivo or in vitro of cells with USPIO contrast agent and tracking of their migration to the target organ in vivo by MRI could be an important tool for understanding the physiologic mechanisms of the CNS in vivo under both normal and pathologic circumstances [33].

In the future, research will aim at evaluating whather such labeled cells may be used further as novel therapeutic CNS tissue-specific drug carriers. The contrast agent marker would confirm that the CNS target has been reached. These specific cell labeling strategies could bring about important progress in cell therapy and in monitoring its efficacy. Another possibility is molecular imaging, which today is still under evaluation by nuclear medicine techniques, but may soon be included among MRI techniques under particular conditions [34].

Conclusions

All published studies in humans or experimental work using dextran-coated iron oxide particles for cell-specific labeling that can be visualized by MRI demonstrate that this approach provides increased diagnostic efficacy for tumors and ischemic brain injury. In inflammatory brain lesions of MS patients, the differences between the classical MRI contrast agent gadolinium and MRI using USPIO provide new functional data on the immunologic reaction of the CNS. As our knowledge of the cell biology of neurodegenerative and CNS inflammatory diseases increases, in vivo cell-specific labeling visualized by MRI is becoming important to evaluate disease activity, to establish prognostic markers, and to monitor treatments and develop new strategies for cell therapy.

Acknowledgements. Our work is supported by ARSEP, LFSEP, Laboratoire Guerbet, Conseil Régional d'Aquitaine, and CNRS-INSERM grant Imagérie du petit animal.

References

1. Filippi M, Grossman RI (2002) MRI techniques to monitor MS evolution. The present and the future. Neurology 58:1147-1153
2. Schoepf U, Marecos EM, Melder RJ et al (1998) Intracellular magnetic labeling of lymphocytes for in vivo trafficking studies. Biotechniques 24:642-651
3. Weissleder R, Cheng HC, Bogdanova A, Bogdanova A Jr (1997) Magnetically labeled cells can be detected be MR imaging. J Magn Reson Imaging 7:258-263
4. Weissleder R (2001) A clearer vision for in vivo imaging. Nat Biotechnol 19:316-317
5. Weissleder R, Elizondo G, Wittenberg J et al (1990) Ultrasmall superparamagnetic iron oxide: characterization of a new class of contrast agents for MR imaging. Radiology 175:489-493
6. Lee S, Weissleder R, Brady T, Wittenberg J (1991) Lymph nodes: microstructural anatomy at MR imaging. Radiology 178:519-522
7. Weissleder R, Heautot JF, Schaffer BK et al (1994) MR lymphography: study of a high-efficiency lymphotropic agent. Radiology 191:225-230
8. Harisinghani MG, Saini S, Weissleder R et al (1999) MR lymphography using ultrasmall superparamagnetic iron oxide in patients with primary abdominal and pelvic malignancies: radiographic-pathologic correlation. AJR Am J Roentol 172:1347-1351
9. Lassmann H, Brück W, Lucchinetti C (2001) Heterogeneity of multiple sclerosis pathogenesis: implications for diagnosis and therapy. Trends Mol Med 7:115-121
10. Dousset V, Delalande C, Ballarino L et al (1999) In vivo macrophage activity imaging in the central nervous system detected by magnetic resonance. Magn Reson Med 41:329-333
11. Dousset V, Ballarino L, Delalande C et al (1999) Comparison of ultrasmall particles of iron oxide (USPIO) T2-weighted, conventional T2-weighted and gadolinium-enhanced T1-weighted MR images in rats with experimental autoimmune encephalomyelitis. AJNR Am J Neuroradiol 20:223-227
12. Dousset V, Gomez C, Petry KG et al (1999) Dose and scanning delay using USPIO for central nervous system macrophage imaging. MAGMA 8:185-189
13. Dousset V, Brochet B, Caillé JM, Petry KG (2000) MS lesions enhancement with ultra small particle iron oxide: the first phase II study. Rev Neurol (Paris) 156(Suppl 3):40
14. Xu S, Jordan EK, Brocke S et al (1998) Study of relapsing remitting experimental aller-

gic encephalomyelitis SJL mouse model using MION-46L enhanced in vivo MRI: early histopathological correlation. J Neurosci Res 52:549-558

15. Doerfler A, Engelhorn T, Heiland S et al (2000) MR contrast agents in acute experimental cerebral ischemia: potential adverse impacts on neurologic outcome and infarction size. J Magn Reson Imaging 11:418-424

16. Rausch M, Baumann D, Neubacher U, Rudin M (2002) In-vivo visualization of phagocytotic cells in rat brains after transient ischemia by USPIO. NMR Biomed 15:278-283

17. Rausch M, Sauter A, Frohlich J et al (2001) Dynamic patterns of USPIO enhancement can be observed in macrophages after ischemic brain damage. Magn Reson Med 46:1018-1022

18. Enochs WS, Harsh G, Hochberg F, Weissleder R (1999) Improved delineation of human brain tumors on MR imaging using long-circulating, superparamagnetic iron oxide agent. J Magn Reson Imaging 9:228-232

19. Varallyay P, Nesbit G, Muldoon LL et al (2002) Comparison of two superparamagnetic viral-sized iron oxide particles ferumoxides and ferumoxtran-10 with a gadolinium chelate in imaging intracranial tumors. AJNR Am J Neuroradiol 23:510-519.

20. Fleige G, Nolte C, Synowitz M et al (2001) Magnetic labeling of activated microglia in experimental gliomas. Neoplasia 3:489-499

21. Gage F, Christen Y (eds) (1997) Isolation, characterization and utilization of CNS stem cells. Springer, Berlin Heidelberg New York

22. Bjornons CRR, Rietze RL, Reynolds BA et al (1999) Turning brain into blood: a hematopoietic fate adopted by adult neural stem cells in vivo. Science 283:534-537

23. Eglitis M, Mezey E (1997) Hematopoietic cells differentiate into both microglia and macroglia in the brains of adult mice. Proc Natl Acad Sci USA 94:4080-4085

24. Sanchez-Ramos J, Song S, Cardozo-Pelaez F et al (2000) Adult bone marrow stromal cells differentiate into neurons in vitro. Exp Neurol 164:247-256

25. Woodburry D, Schwartz EJ, Prockop DJ, Black IB (2000) Adult rat and human bone marrow stromal cells differentiate into neurons. J Neurosci Rev 61:364-370

26. Kopen GC, Prockop DJ, Phinney DG (1999) Marrow stromal cells migrate throughout forebrain and cerebellum, and they differentiate into astrocytes after injection into neonatal mouse brains. Proc Natl Acad Sci USA 96:10711-10716

27. Mezey E, Chandross KJ, Harta G et al (2000) Turning blood into brain: cells bearing neuronal antigens generated in vivo from bone marrow. Science 290:1779-1782

28. Bulte JW, Zhang S, van Gelderen P et al (1999) Neurotransplantation of magnetically labeled oligodendrocyte progenitors: MR tracking of cell migration and myelination. Proc Natl Acad Sci USA 96: 15256-15261

29. Bulte JWM, Duncan ID, Frank JA (2002) In vivo magnetic resonance tracking of magnetically labeled cells after transplantation. J Cereb Blood Flow Metab 22:899-907

30. Doche de Laquitane B, Dousset V, Solanilla A et al (2002) Iron particle labelling of haemopoietic progenitor cells: an in vitro study. Biosci Rep (in press)

31. Sipe JC, Filippi M, Martino G et al (1999) Method for intracellular magnetic labeling of human mononuclear cells using approved iron contrast agents. Magn Reson Imaging 17:1521-1523

32. Lewin M, Carlesso N, Tung CH et al (2000) Tat peptide-derivatized magnetic nanoparticles allows in vivo tracking and recovery of progenitor cells. Nat Biotechnol 18:410-414

33. Schoepf U, Marecos EM, Melder RJ et al (1998) Intracellular magnetic labeling of lymphocytes for in vivo trafficking studies. Biotechniques 24:642-651

34. Weissleder R (1999) Molecular imaging: exploring the next frontier. Radiology 212:609-614

Chapter 2

Magnetization Transfer Imaging

M. Rovaris, M. Filippi

Introduction

In multiple sclerosis (MS), conventional magnetic resonance (MR) imaging (MRI) has proved to be sensitive for detecting disease-related abnormalities and their changes over time [1]. However, conventional MRI is not able to provide accurate estimates of the extent and nature of the associated tissue damage. Quantitative MR-based techniques, with increased pathological specificity to the heterogeneous substrates of central nervous system (CNS) pathology, have the potential to overcome these limitations. Among these techniques, magnetization transfer imaging (MTI) has been one of the most extensively applied to the assessment of MS, in part because of its ability to detect and quantify microstructural damage in tissues which appear normal on conventional MR images [2]. The present chapter will outline the major contributions of MTI to the study of MS pathobiology.

Basic Principles of MTI

MT contrast is used in a number of applications in MRI [3] and results from the interactions between the protons in free fluid in a tissue and those protons found in macromolecules. While the magnetization from these macromolecules cannot be observed directly, proton magnetization is in constant exchange between the free fluid and the macromolecules, and so magnetization saturation and relaxation within the macromolecule affects the observable signal from the free water [4].

MT contrast is achieved by applying radiofrequency (RF) power only to the proton magnetization of the macromolecules. Since in brain tissue the free water protons and macromolecular protons have the same central resonance frequency but very different line widths, this can be achieved by shifting the frequency of the saturating RF pulses to one side of the free water resonance line [5]. The RF pulse frequency offset is chosen to minimize direct saturation of the free pool, while remaining small enough not to be out of the frequency range of the broad resonance line of the macromolecular spins.

The most general description of the MT effect uses data acquired at a range of saturating powers and offsets, and models the system as two or more compartments [6]. This allows both the relaxation rates of the pools and their relative proportions to be determined. More simply, the MT effect can be characterized by a nonspecific pseudo rate constant (k_f) for the MT process, where it should be noted that k_f includes both chemical exchange and dipolar coupling between bound and free protons. k_f can be found by measuring the free water signal twice: once in the presence and once in the absence of the MT saturating pulses. The free water relaxation rate in the presence of the saturating pulses (R_{1sat}) must also be measured, in which case:

$$k_f = R_{1sat} \frac{(M_0 \pm M_s)}{M_0},$$

where M_0 is the magnitude of the free water proton signal in the absence of the off-resonance saturating pulses, and M_s is the magnitude of the free water proton signal with the off-resonance saturating pulses applied. Note, however, that the above equation is only strictly valid in the case of perfect saturation of the bound pool, a condition that cannot be achieved in vivo on clinical scanners. If the rate constant is not specifically of interest, then we can form the MT ratio (MTR), a simple measure of MT effects:

$$\text{MTR} \frac{(M_0 \pm M_s)}{M_0} \, 100\%.$$

Low MTR indicates a reduced capacity of free water to exchange magnetization with the brain tissue matrix with which the water comes into intimate contact. For example, in cerebrospinal fluid (CSF), where there is an almost complete absence of macromolecules, no exchange can occur, the observable signal is unaffected by the saturation pulses, and the MTR approaches zero. In healthy brain tissue, where M_s drops significantly below M_0 as the saturated magnetization is transferred to the observable water, an MTR of up to 40-50% may be seen, depending on the pulse sequence used.

Pathological Basis of MTI Changes in MS

In MS lesions, a reduction of MTR values may be caused either by a reduction in the integrity of the macromolecular matrix, reflecting damage to the myelin or to the axonal membrane [7], or by dilution of the macromolecules by inflammatory edema [7]. Studies with animal models [8, 9] reported that MTR drops only slightly with edema but more strongly with severe demyelination and axonal loss. A marked reduction of MTR has been found in a primate model of lysolecithin-induced demyelination [9], in a feline model of wallerian degeneration [10], and in regions with pathologically proven axonal damage following experimental brain trauma in the pig [11]. Markedly reduced MTR values are also measured in the "pure" demyelinating lesions of patients with progressive multifocal leukoencephalopathy (PML) [12, 13] or central pontine myelinolysis [14], and in the affected optic nerves of patients with optic neuritis, where it correlated with increased latency of the visual evoked potentials [15], the increased latency being itself related to the extent and severity of demyelination. Follow-up studies in primates affected by relapsing experimental allergic encephalomyelitis demonstrated that, after MTR reduction in the acute phase of lesion development, it is possible to observe recoveries of MTR [16].

This temporal profile of the MTR might correlate with demyelination and remyelination during lesion development and resolution [16]. The influence of remyelination on MTR values is confirmed by a study of the corpus callosum of rats with lysophosphatidylcholine-induced demyelination, which is known to remyelinate spontaneously [17]. In this study [17], the recovery of MTR values after their initial decrease was significantly associated with an increasing number of remyelinating axons. The relationship between reduced MTR values and axonal loss is suggested by the strong correlation found in MS lesions between MTR and N-acetylaspartate (NAA) levels [18] (NAA is an MR spectroscopy marker of axonal dysfunction [19]), signal intensity on T1-weighted images [20], and mean diffusivity [21]. An association between MTR and axonal density is also indirectly confirmed by the demonstration of markedly reduced MTR values in the optic nerves of patients with Leber's hereditary optic neuropathy [22]. However, the most compelling evidence that marked MTR reduction corresponds to severe tissue damage comes from a postmortem study of lesions and normal-appearing white matter (NAWM) from patients with MS [23]. In this study, strong correlations were found between MTR and the percentage of residual axons and the degree of demyelination.

Methodological Aspects of MTI Analysis

After the creation of MT-calculated maps, where the signal intensity is related to MTR values of individual pixels, several approaches can be used to analyze MS-related abnormalities:

1. *Region of interest (ROI) analysis*. This approach allows the study of individual MS lesions and discrete areas of the NAWM and gray matter.
2. *Analysis of the average MTR of T2-visible lesions*. This approach allows information to be obtained about the severity of tissue damage of the overall lesion population. The average lesion MTR can be computed, as

$$\text{average lesion MTR} = \frac{\sum_i A_i \times \text{MTR}_i}{\sum_i A_i},$$

where A_i is the area of lesion i, and MTR_i is the average MTR within that lesion. Thus the contribution that each lesion makes to the average is weighted by the size of the lesion.
3. *Contour plotting*. This approach consists in displaying the MTR values as an

overlay on MR images [24, 25]. In this way, it is possible to detect gradients and boundaries of abnormal MTR that are too subtle to be detected by conventional reading of the MTR maps.

4. *Histogram analysis.* This strategy encompasses both micro- and macrostructural damage in the examined tissue [26]. The first step in the creation of the histogram is a preliminary manual or semiautomated image segmentation aimed at excluding all the extraparenchymal tissues. Secondly, to reduce the effects of image noise and also CSF signal, all the pixels with very low MTR (i.e., from 0 to 5-10%) are also excluded from the analysis. Then, the data set of MTR values is displayed as a histogram, which is usually normalized to the total number of pixels to allow comparisons of histograms from subjects with different brain or cord size. For each histogram, several parameters can be calculated. These include the height and position of the histogram peak (i.e., the most common MTR value in the brain), the average MTR, and the MTR corresponding to the 25th, 50th, and 75th percentiles of the histogram (MTR_{25}, MTR_{50}, and MTR_{75}), that indicate the MTR at which the integral of the histogram is 25%, 50%, and 75% of the total, respectively. MTR histogram analysis is a highly automated technique and, as a consequence, the intra-rater, inter-rater and scan-rescan variabilities of MTR histogram-derived metrics are low [27, 28].

MTI Studies of Individual MS Lesions

In MS, MRI-visible lesions enhancing after Gd injection represent areas with a damaged BBB and ongoing inflammation [29, 30]. However, "active" MS lesions may have different patterns (e.g., homogeneous or ring-like) or different durations of enhancement [29], or may enhance only when highly sensitive approaches are used, such as the administration of a triple dose of Gd [31]. This variability in enhancement suggests that the pathological nature of enhancing MS lesions and the severity of the associated changes in the inflamed tissue may vary widely. MTI studies of individual enhancing lesions confirmed this perception. Homogeneously enhancing lesions, which may represent new active lesions, have significantly higher MTR values than ring-enhancing lesions [32-35], which may represent old, reactivated lesions. In the latter lesions, the central portions, which probably represent the most damaged tissue, have the lowest MTR values [35]. A longitudinal study [36] has also confirmed that ring-like enhancing lesions had the lowest MTR, both at baseline and at follow-up, after enhancement ceased. The duration of enhancement is also associated with different degrees of MTR changes in new MS lesions: lesions enhancing on at least two consecutive monthly scans have lower MTRs than those enhancing on a single scan [37]. This indicates that longer enhancement in MS lesions may be related to more severe tissue damage. That a less disrupted BBB is associated with milder tissue damage is also indicated by the demonstration that new lesions enhancing after the injection of a standard dose of Gd have significantly lower

MTR values than those enhancing only after a triple dose [38], and that large enhancing lesions tend to have greater MTR reductions than smaller lesions [32].

Using MTI and variable frequencies of scanning, several authors have investigated the structural changes of new enhancing MS lesions for periods of time ranging from 3 to 36 months [32, 36, 38-45]. The results of all these studies consistently show that, on average, MTR drops dramatically when the lesions start to enhance and may show a partial or complete recovery in the subsequent 1-6 months. However, only three of these studies [36, 43, 45] evaluated the evolution of individual lesions in an attempt to define the prevalence of lesions whose MTR values remain stable, or improve, or worsen during the follow-up, and found that only a minority of the enhancing lesions from patients with mildly disabling forms of MS have progressive structural damage soon after their formation. New lesions enhancing only after the injection of a triple dose of Gd have a similar short-term MTR recovery profile to those enhancing after a standard dose [38]. However, at each time point of the follow-up, MTR in triple-dose-enhancing lesions is significantly higher than in standard-dose-enchancing lesions [38]. This again confirms the relative mildness of tissue damage in those lesions with less severe BBB disruption.

These results suggest that the balance between damaging and reparative mechanisms may be highly variable during the early phases of MS lesion formation. Different proportions of lesions with different degrees of structural changes may, therefore, contribute to the evolution of the disease and may explain why previous studies found poor correlations between the number of enhancing lesions and the long-term disease evolution [46]. In a patient at presentation with an isolated lesion of the type seen in MS, it was shown that there was a strict relationship between the MTR recovery in this newly formed lesion located in the internal capsule and the corresponding recovery of the contralateral sensorimotor deficit [42]. A recent 3-year follow-up study [44] showed that newly enhancing lesions from patients with secondary progressive MS (SPMS) compared to those from patients with relapsing-remitting MS (RRMS) had lower MTR at the time of their appearance and presented a more severe and significant MTR reduction during the follow-up.

MTR values for MS lesions visible on T2-weighted scans are significantly lower than those for NAWM [33, 47-50] and those of lesions from elderly patients [51] or from patients with small-vessel disease [49], systemic immune-mediated diseases [52], human immunodeficiency virus (HIV) encephalitis [12], CNS tuberculosis [53], traumatic brain injury [25], or migraine [54]. In contrast, reductions of MTR values of a magnitude comparable to that seen in MS lesions have been found in white matter lesions of patients with vascular dementia [55], amyotrophic lateral sclerosis [56], PML [12, 13], central pontine myelinolysis [14], cerebral autosomal dominant arteriopathy with subcortical infarcts and leukoencephalopathy (CADASIL) [57], Laber's hereditary optic neuropathy [22], and acute disseminated encephalomyelitis [58]. Nevertheless, regardless of the average lesion MTR values found in all these conditions, the lesions of MS tend to have a greater variability of their MTR values, perhaps as a consequence of their wider temporal and pathological heterogeneity.

Lower MTR has been reported in hypointense MS lesions than in lesions that are isointense to NAWM on T1-weighted scans [34-36], and MTR has been found to be inversely correlated with the degree of hypointensity [34, 59]. In a longitudinal study [36] with monthly MTI and T1-weighted scans, van Waesberghe et al. found that MS lesions that changed from hypointense to isointense when Gd enhancement ceased also had a significant MTR increase, whereas a strongly decreased MTR at the time of initial enhancement was predictive of a persistent T1-weighted hypointensity and lower MTR after 6 months. On the basis of these results and of a postmortem study [23], it may be argued that "fixed" MS lesions with lower MTR are expressions of more severe demyelination and axonal loss.

Decreased MTR has also been found for NAWM areas that are adjacent to focal T2-visible MS lesions [47, 48, 50]. MTR progressively increased with distance from MS lesions to the cortical gray matter (GM), and was lower for patients with more disabling MS courses [47]. The latter findings suggest that the actual size of MS lesions is greater than the size visible on T2-weighted images, and that the demyelinating "penumbra" detected by MTI might be relevant in determining patients' disability.

That average lesion MTR may give information on MS tissue damage additional to that provided by other MRI measures of disease burden is suggested by the weak correlations reported between average lesion MTR and lesion load or brain volume [60, 61]. The moderate correlations that have been found between average lesion MTR and other measures of intrinsic lesion damage derived from diffusion tensor (DT) MRI [21, 50, 61] and MR spectroscopy [18, 62], albeit stronger than those with MRI measures of macroscopic MS disease burden, also support this concept. Even though the average lesion MTR was found to be the best discriminant between patients with MS and those with CNS symptoms or signs of systemic immune-mediated disorders, independently of the burden of MRI-visible lesions [52], the correlations between average lesion MTR and the clinical manifestations of MS are somewhat disappointing [60, 61]. Patients with cognitive impairment have a significantly lower average lesion MTR than those without, but average lesion MTR was found to explain only 35% of the total variance in neuropsychological test performance [63].

Similar average lesion MTR values have been found in patients with SPMS and primary progressive MS (PPMS) matched for the degree of disability [64]. Consistent with their clinical evolution, patients with SPMS show a faster decline in their average MTR values than those with any of the other clinical phenotypes of the disease [65]. Average lesion MTR was found to be lower in patients with RRMS than in those presenting with clinically isolated syndromes (CIS) suggestive of MS, but in the latter group of patients it did not predict subsequent disease evolution [66]. Also, average lesion MTR was not found to differ significantly between patients with RRMS and those with benign MS or SPMS [67], nor between patients with and those without fatigue [68]. The only partial correlation found between the degree of intrinsic lesion damage as measured using average lesion MTR and the clinical manifestations of MS might be due, on the one hand, to the variable extent of tissue damage outside T2-visible lesions and, on the other, by the fact that intrinsic lesion damage can induce adaptive cortical changes [69], which in turn have the potential to limit the clinical consequences of subcortical white matter damage [69-72].

MTI Studies of Microstructural MS Damage

Postmortem studies show that abnormalities can be detected in the NAWM from patients with MS [73, 74]. These abnormalities include diffuse astrocytic hyperplasia, patchy edema, and perivascular cellular infiltration. In addition, Arstila et al. described abnormally thin myelin in biopsies from NAWM of MS patients [75], and two recent postmortem studies also detected signs of axonal damage in MS NAWM [76, 77]. Such pathological abnormalities modify the relative proportions of mobile and immobile protons in the diseased tissue, and therefore it is not surprising that MTI is able to show microstructural damage in the NAWM that is not detected by conventional imaging [47, 48, 50].

Variable degrees of NAWM changes may precede new lesion formation in MS [39, 40, 78]. Edema, marked astrocytic proliferation, perivascular inflammation, and demyelination all may account for an increased amount of unbound water and, as a consequence, determine MTR changes prior to the appearance of T2-visible abnormalities.

Several ROI-based studies have shown that NAWM MTR reductions are invariably detected in all the major phenotypes of MS and are diffuse in several cerebral regions [47, 48, 50]. Decreased MTR values have been found in several NAWM regions even in patients with clinically definite MS and no or only very few T2-visible lesions [79]. In a recent longitudinal study [80], the average NAWM MTR of patients with RRMS and SPMS yielded a positive predictive value of about 78% for the clinical evolution of the disease after 5 years, suggesting that the MTI assessment of microstructural brain changes might become a useful tool for the monitoring of MS treatment.

The need to obtain more comprehensive estimates of the overall extent of NAWM damage in MS has led to the application of histogram analysis to all brain pixels classed as normal on conventional MRI [81]. This approach requires the prior identification of macroscopic lesions on T2-weighted images, the outlines of which are then superimposed onto the coregistered MTR maps and nulled out, thus obtaining MTR maps of normal-appearing brain tissue (NABT). Using an approach of this kind, Tortorella et al. [81] showed that NABT MTR histogram abnormalities are present in all the main MS clinical phenotypes, and are more pronounced in patients with SPMS. In RRMS patients, average MTR of the NABT was found to be highly correlated with cognitive impairment [63], but not with the severity of fatigue [68]. Interestingly, a recent study of a large cohort of patients has shown that the NABT MTR histogram characteristics of patients with PPMS do not significantly differ from those of patients with SPMS with similar levels of disability, even though patients with SPMS had higher T2-visible lesion burdens [64]. A significant decline of NABT MTR over time has been shown to occur at a faster pace in patients with SPMS than in patients with other clinical phenotypes [65]. Reduced MTR values have also been detected in the NABT from patients at presentation with CIS, and the extent of these abnormalities has been found to be an independent predictor of subsequent disease evolution [66]. These findings, however, have not been confirmed by other investigators using ROI [82] or whole-brain histogram [83] analysis. More recently, subtle, but significant, NABT MTR histogram changes have also been discovered in first-degree relatives of patients with MS compared to healthy controls from a general population [84]. In MS patients, NABT MTR values are only partially correlated with the extent of macroscopic lesions and the severity of intrinsic lesion damage, suggesting that NABT changes do not only reflect wallerian degeneration of axons traversing large focal abnormalities [61, 64, 81].

The correlation between MTI and DT MRI-derived metrics thought to reflect NAWM or NABT damage has been found to be weak to moderate in strength [21, 50, 61]. This suggests that brain damage occurring in the absence of conventional MRI-detectable abnormalities is the result of a complex relationship between destructive and reparative mechanisms, which may have variable effects on MT and DT MRI findings. More recently, in patients with RRMS [69] and PPMS [72], moderate to strong correlations have also been found between the severity of structural changes of the NABT (as measured using MTI) and the relative activations of several cortical areas located in a widespread network for sensorimotor and multimodal integration, measured using functional MRI. This suggests that not only macroscopic MS lesions, but also subtle NABT changes can cause adaptive cortical reorganization with the potential to limit the functional consequences of MS-related structural damage.

The role of NAWM MTR changes in the diagnostic work-up of patients suspected of having MS remains to be elucidated, but it is likely to be modest, since these changes are not disease-specific. Indeed, reduced NAWM MTR values can also be found in patients with other neurological conditions associated with nonspecific white matter lesions on T2-weighted images, such as neuro-SLE [85] (Fig. 1), CADASIL [57], PML [12], HIV-encephalitis [12], Leber's hereditary optic neuropathy [22], and head trauma [25]. Nevertheless, it might be worth noting that MTR changes of the NAWM have not been found in patients with other conditions, such as migraine and multiple T2 lesions [54], Devic's neuromyelitis optica [86], and acute disseminated encephalomyelitis [58], which can also be considered in the differential diagnosis of patients with MS.

Using NABT histogram analysis, it is not possible to define the relative contributions of NAWM and GM pathology to the observed changes. Nevertheless, NAWM represents the largest part of the NABT included in MTR histograms and, as a consequence, it is likely that the major contribution comes from subtle white matter abnormalities rather than from abnormalities in the GM. Consistent with this, preliminary data coming from histogram analysis of NAWM taken in isolation confirmed those obtained from the analysis of the NABT [85, 87]. However,

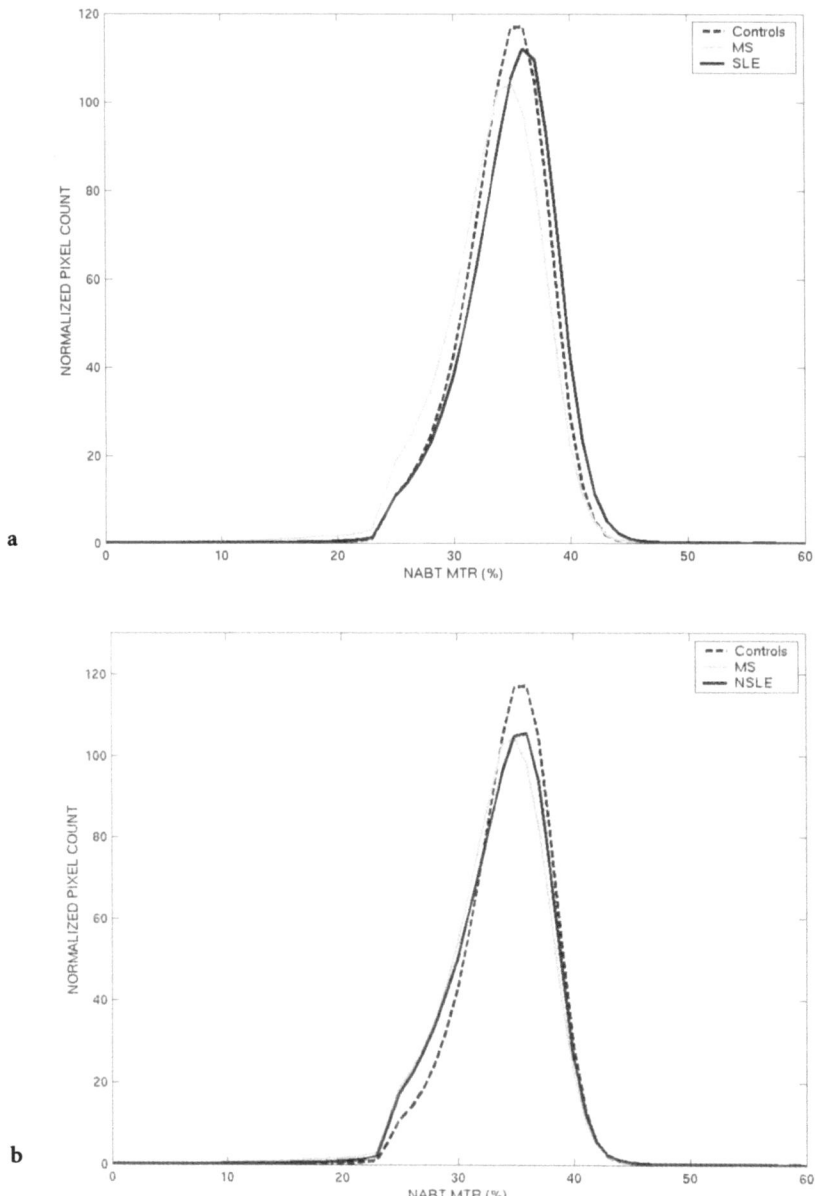

Fig. 1. NABT MTR histograms from healthy controls, patients with RRMS, patients with systemic lupus erythematosus (SLE) without clinical signs of neurological involvement (**a**), or patients with neuropsychiatric SLE (NSLE) (**b**). For SLE patients, the shape of the histogram resembles that of healthy controls and average NABT MTR values are significantly higher than those of MS patients. On the other hand, there are no significant differences between MS and NSLE patients in terms of NABT MTR histogram-derived metrics, as reflected by the similar shape of the histograms from the two groups

postmortem studies have shown that MS pathology does not spare cerebral GM [88, 89]. Consistent with this, recent studies have shown reduced MTR values in the GM from patients with MS, using ROI [85] or histogram [85, 87, 90] analysis. Interestingly, in one study [90] the peak height of the GM MTR histogram was inversely correlated with the severity of clinical disability ($r = -0.65$). Cortical/subcortical brain tissue MTR [91], but not basal ganglia MTR [92], was found to differ significantly between MS patients and healthy controls and to correlate strongly with MS cognitive impairment [91]. However, GM MTR histograms were not different between patients with and those without fatigue [93]. Significant correlations have also been reported between GM MTR histographic changes and T2-visible lesion volume [85, 90]. This fits with the notion that at least part of GM pathology in MS is secondary to retrograde degeneration of fibers traversing white matter lesions.

MTI Studies of Overall MS Brain Damage

Consistently with the evidence that the extent and nature of the damage T2-visible abnormalities, NAWM and GM all contribute to the accumulation of irreversible neurological disability in MS, there has been increasing use of MR metrics with the potential to provide a complete assessment of MS pathology in the brain. One of the simplest and most robust approaches is the production of MTR histograms of the whole of the brain tissue. However, this approach is not without limitations. First, by constructing an MTR histogram, one gives up the spatial information present in an image and instead looks at the distribution of MTR values. Second, the cerebral atrophy that occurs in MS [94, 59] can lead to an increase in the contamination of the signal from parenchyma by signal from CSF. This is particularly difficult to account for, since although a simple intensity cut-off to remove the CSF signal will ameliorate the problem, partial volume effects mean that it is not possible to set the cut-off to remove the effect of CSF completely.

Due to the presence of diffuse demyelination and axonal loss, MS patients typically have lower whole-brain average MTR, as well as lower peak height and position of the whole-brain MTR histogram than normal subjects [21, 26, 64, 65, 67, 96, 97]. MTR histogram parameters also differ between the various clinical forms of MS [65, 67, 96, 97]. Typically, patients with SPMS have the lowest whole-brain MTR histogram-derived measures [64, 67, 96, 97]. In patients with SPMS, whole-brain MTR histogram metrics also appear to be particularly sensitive to disease changes over relatively short periods of time [65]. This exquisite sensitivity could make these quantities appealing as outcome measures for assessing the efficacy of experimental treatments in patients with SPMS. Preliminary work has also suggested a potential role of whole-brain MTR histograms in the diagnostic work-up of individual MS cases, especially in the absence of "typical" conventional MRI changes [98].

Correlations between MTR histogram parameters and clinical outcome have been widely tested [21, 26, 60, 61, 64, 65, 67, 96, 97, 99-101]. Moderate to strong cor-

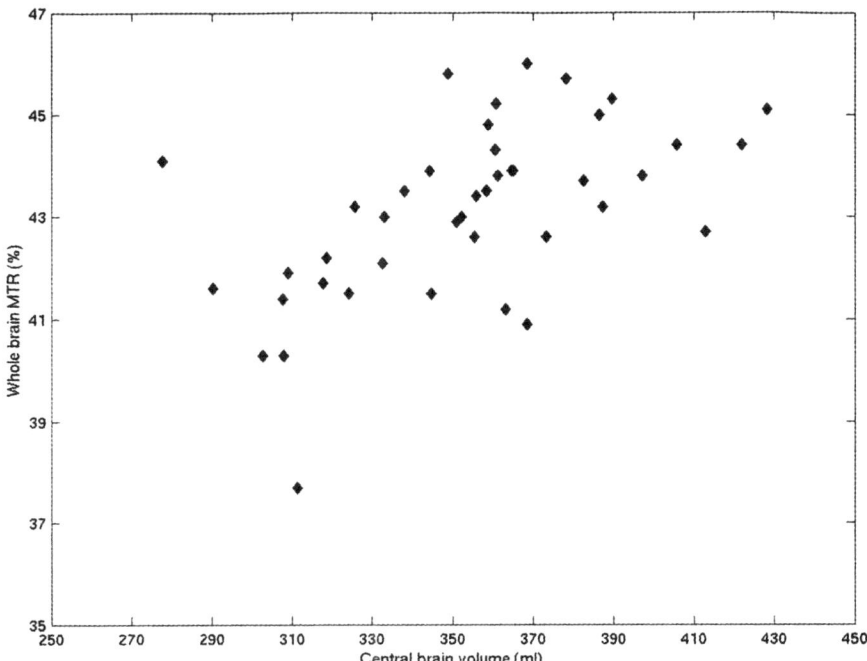

Fig. 2. Scatterplot of the values of average whole-brain MTR versus those of absolute central brain tissue volume (as measured from a slab of contiguous periventricular axial slices) in patients with RRMS or SPMS. A significant correlation exists between the two measures ($r = 0.57$), indicating that part of the variability of whole-brain MTR histogram-derived metrics can be explained by the severity of MS-related neurodegenerative processes

relations between various whole-brain MTR histogram-derived metrics and the severity of physical disability have been confirmed by various of these studies [96, 97, 100]. Whole-brain MTR/clinical correlations were found to be stronger in patients with RRMS and SPMS than in other clinical phenotypes of the disease [96, 97], while no significant correlations were found when patients with PPMS were considered in isolation [64, 96, 97]. Whole-brain MTR histogram metrics are also correlated with the presence of neuropsychological impairment in MS patients [99, 102, 103].

Several studies [26, 60, 61, 97, 104] suggest that MTR histogram parameters in MS patients are influenced not only by the lesion burden in cerebral tissues, but also by the volume of brain parenchyma (Fig. 2). Van Buchem et al. [26] found that the absolute (i.e., not corrected for differences in brain volume between individuals) MTR histogram peak height is largely influenced by the total volume of pixels entering the analysis. In the same study [26], the relative (i.e., normalized for brain volumes) MTR histogram peak height was highly correlated with average brain MTR, MTR_{25}, and MTR_{50}, but not with MTR_{75}. This indicates that, in MS patients, a lowering of the relative histogram peak height reflects a decrease in the amount of brain tissue with truly normal MTR. Phillips et al. [104] found strong inverse correlations between MTR histogram peak height and both T2-weighted lesion volume ($r = -0.73$) and CSF volume ($r = -0.83$), and a positive correlation between T2-weighted lesion volume and CSF volume ($r = 0.73$). In another MTI study of 42 MS patients [60], significant correlations were found between T2-weighted lesion load and brain tissue MTR, histogram peak height, MTR_{25}, and MTR_{50}; and between T1-weighted lesion load and average lesion MTR, brain tissue MTR, MTR_{25}, and MTR_{50}. Brain volume correlated significantly with many of the above-mentioned MTI measures. Kalkers et al. [97] selectively investigated the subgroup of MTR histogram parameters more closely related to partial volume averaging effects from enlarged CSF spaces. They found that these so-called CSF-related MTR variables (reflecting the lower left portion of brain MTR histograms) were distinguishing SPMS patients from healthy controls and those with other MS phenotypes better than parenchymal variables, underpinning the role played by brain atrophy in determining MS-related changes of brain MTR histograms. That this role is especially relevant in the more disabling and advanced phases of MS is also suggested by the lack of significant correlations between brain volume and MTR histogram metrics found by Iannucci et al. [61] in a sample of RRMS patients with mild disease severity.

MTI Studies of the Cervical Cord and Optic Nerve

MTI of the cervical cord and optic nerve presents technical difficulties, mainly because of the size of these two structures and their tendency to move during imaging. Nevertheless, recent work has shown that it is possible to acquire good-quality MT images of the cervical cord [105] and optic nerve [15, 106]. Cervical cord and optic nerves are attractive regions in which to study the pathophysiology of MS. Thus, the application of MTI to the assessment of MS-related damage in these structures is likely to increase our understanding of the mechanisms leading to the development of irreversible disability in MS.

Preliminary studies [107, 108] using ROI analysis and small cohorts of patients found that the cervical cord of MS patients had lower MTR values than that of controls. More recently, the contribution made by the cervical cord to the clinical manifestations of MS has been studied using MTR histogram analysis [109]. The entire cohort of patients with MS had significantly lower average MTR of the overall cervical cord tissue than control subjects. Compared to control subjects, patients with RRMS had similar cervical cord MTR histogram-derived measures, whereas those with with PPMS had significantly lower average MTR and peak height. Patients with SPMS had lower MTR histogram peak height than those with RRMS. The peak height and position of the cervical cord MTR histogram were independent predictors of the probability of having locomotor disability. A more recent study has compared cervical cord MTR histogram metrics of

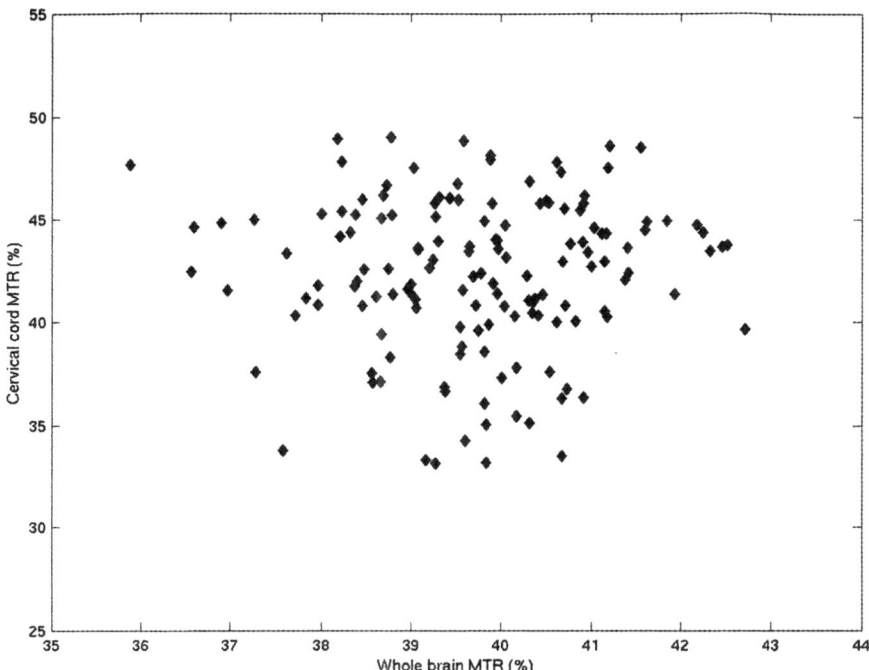

Fig. 3. Scatterplot of the values of average whole-brain MTR versus those of average cervical cord MTR in patients with PPMS or SPMS. There is no significant correlation between
these parameters. This indicates that MS pathology in the cord is not a mere reflection of
brain pathology, and that MTI studies of the brain and cervical cord can provide complementary information on the actual disease burden

patients with PPMS and SPMS and found no significant difference between these
two groups [64]. In PPMS, a model including cord area and cord MTR histogram
peak height was significantly, albeit modestly, associated with the level of disability. No or only moderate correlations have been found between brain T2-visible
lesion load [109] or average brain MTR [110] and cervical cord MTR histogram
metrics (Fig. 3). This suggests that MS pathology in the cord is not a mere reflection of brain pathology (as it is in other conditions such as CADASIL) [111].
Another study [86] found no significant difference between any of the cervical
cord MTR histogram metrics of patients with MS and Devic's neuromyelitis optica, despite the fact that the macroscopic lesions in the cervical cord of the latter
patients were longer and had a conventional MRI appearance suggesting more
severe intrinsic damage than those of the MS patients. This again suggests the relevance of subtle changes in the NAWM of patients with MS [76].

Thorpe et al. [15] measured MTR of the optic nerves of 20 MS patients with
optic neuritis. They found significant differences in MTR between affected nerves
and both unaffected nerves and controls. In the affected nerves MTR correlated

with the length of the lesions visible on T2-weighted scans and with visual evoked potential latency, but not with visual acuity and color vision. Boorstein et al. [106] also reported a reduction of MTR values in the affected nerve of patients with acute unilateral optic neuritis independently of the presence of T2-visible lesions. The asymptomatic nerves had MTR values similar to those from control subjects. More recently, Inglese et al. [112] have shown that MTR of the optic nerves from MS patients with incomplete or no recovery from a previous episode of acute optic neuritis is significantly lower than the corresponding quantities of the optic nerves from MS patients with complete functional recovery after an episode of acute optic neuritis, but not different from those of the optic nerves from patients with Leber's hereditary optic neuropathy. In contrast, MTR values of the affected optic nerves from patients with recovery did not differ from the corresponding quantities in clinically unaffected optic nerves, which had MTR values similar to those of the optic nerves from healthy volunteers [112]. At present, these data are the strongest in vivo evidence that, in patients with MS, neurodegeneration is associated with functional deficits secondary to incomplete recovery from relapses.

Use of MTI to Monitor MS Treatment Efficacy

Recent guidelines from the White Matter Study Group of the International Society for Magnetic Resonance in Medicine recommended the use of MTI in the context of large-scale MS trials as an adjunctive measure to monitor disease evolution [113], mainly for the following reasons. First, MTI can provide quantitative metrics with some specificity to MS-related irreversible tissue loss. Second, it enables us to assess the entire brain, an important aspect considering that MS is a widespread disease affecting all the CNS tissues. Third, quantities derived from MTI are reproducible, correlated with the degree of disability and cognitive impairment, sensitive to disease changes, and relatively cost-effective (high-quality data can be obtained with a scanning time of less than 10 min).

Only preliminary data have been published regarding the effects of available disease-modifying treatments for MS on MTI-derived parameters [114-116]. All these studies were conducted in small sample sizes and with a baseline-versus-treatment design. Two of them have shown that treatment with interferon beta-1b [115] or interferon beta-1a [116] favorably modifies the recovery of MTR values that follows the cessation of Gd enhancement in newly formed lesions in RRMS patients. On the other hand, Richert et al. [115] did not find any significant difference in the MTR values of NAWM ROIs before and during interferon beta-1b therapy, nor in whole-brain MTR histogram-derived parameters from another cohort of RRMS patients receiving the same treatment regimen [114]. In the latter study, month-to-month fluctuations of the histogram peak height persisted during the treatment period despite the almost complete suppression of contrast-enhanced MRI activity.

At present, MTI has already been used in various phase II and phase III trials for RRMS (injectable and oral interferon beta-1a, interferon beta-1b, and oral glatiramer acetate) and SPMS (interferon beta-1b and immunoglobulins). In all these trials, MTI acquisition has, however, been limited to highly specialized MR centers, and only subgroups of patients (about 50-100 per trial) have therefore been studied. Although the complete results from these MTI studies have not yet been published, preliminary reports [117, 118] from the two SPMS trials indicated a lack of treatment efficacy on MTR histogram-derived parameters, but confirmed that MTI might be sensitive enough to detect disease-related changes over short periods of time.

MTI Studies of MS: Future Developments

Although at present virtually all clinical MTI studies are based on MTR measurements, the reduction of the MT phenomenon to a single MTR value has limited the interpretation of the results and the ability to achieve optimal standardization of MTR measurements across multiple centers. MTI uses off-resonance RF pulses to create contrast, and the MTR values obtained strongly depend on the offset frequency, bandwidth, and average power of the pulses. Differences between sites can be minimized by standardizing the pulse sequence implementation and choice of parameters, although where multiple different scanner types are to be used, this may lead to the use of a "lowest common denominator" sequence rather than an optimal one. An alternative and more promising approach is the application of new methodology to quantify all the observable and physically independent parameters of the MT phenomenon [119]. Recent studies [120, 121] have applied multiparametric MTI sequences to the study of MS and found that metrics such as k_f and fractional pool size are sensitive to changes occurring in the NAWM before lesion appearance [120], allowing us reliably to quantify the extent of tissue disruption within T1 "black holes" [121].

Newer approaches to the interpretation of MTR histograms have also been proposed, based upon linear discriminant analysis (LDA) and principal component analysis (PCA) [101]. LDA might be better applied when using MTR histograms for group classifications, whereas PCA, which seems to limit the effects of the intersubject variability of histogram-derived metrics, may be useful to improve the correlation between histogram characteristics and clinical findings. In patients with PPMS, the use of PCA has yielded a stronger correlation with disability than that seen using standard MTR histogram measurement [122, 123].

Conclusions

Thanks to its increased sensitivity to microstructural tissue changes and specificity to the heterogeneous pathological substrates of MS lesions, MTI can give complementary information to conventional MRI in a noninvasive manner. MTR histograms provide a means of estimating the relative volumes of tissues characterized by specific ranges of MTR, and allow conclusions to be drawn regarding both focal and diffuse aspects of the disease. This indicates the potential of MTI for detecting relevant changes of lesion pathology during experimental treatment of MS patients. Refinements in the techniques and equipment used for the acquisition and postprocessing of MTI should result in more precise measures of the MT effect, and eventually in more specific techniques for noninvasive MR-based evaluation of MS patients.

References

1. Rovaris M, Filippi M (1999) Magnetic resonance techniques to monitor disease evolution and treatment trial outcomes in multiple sclerosis. Curr Opin Neurol 12:337-344
2. Filippi M, Tortorella C, Bozzali M (1999) Normal-appearing-white-matter changes in multiple sclerosis: the contribution of magnetic resonance techniques. Mult Scler 5:273-282
3. Wolff SD, Balaban RS (1994) Magnetization transfer imaging – practical aspects and clinical applications. Radiology 192:593-599
4. Balaban RS, Ceckler TL (1992) Magnetization transfer contrast in magnetic resonance imaging. Magn Reson Q 8:116-137
5. Wolff SD, Balaban RS (1989) Magnetization transfer contrast (MTC) and tissue water proton relaxation in vivo. Magn Reson Med 10:135-144
6. Henkelman RM, Huang XM, Xiang QS et al (1993) Quantitative interpretation of magnetization transfer. Magn Reson Med 29:759-766
7. McDonald WI, Miller DH, Barnes D (1992) The pathological evolution of multiple sclerosis. Neuropathol Appl Neurobiol 18:319-334
8. Dousset V, Grossman RI, Ramer KN et al (1992) Experimental allergic encephalomyelitis and multiple sclerosis: lesion characterization with magnetization transfer imaging [published erratum appears in Radiology 1992;183:878]. Radiology 182:483-491
9. Dousset V, Brochet B, Vital A et al (1995) Lysolecithin-induced demyelination in primates: preliminary in vivo study with MR and magnetization transfer. AJNR Am J Neuroradiol 16:225-231
10. Lexa FJ, Grossman RI, Rosenquist AC (1994) MR of wallerian degeneration in the feline visual system: characterization by magnetization transfer rate with histopathologic correlation. AJNR Am J Neuroradiol 15:201-212
11. Kimura H, Meaney DF, McGowan JC et al (1996) Magnetization transfer imaging of diffuse axonal injury following experimental brain injury in the pig: characterization by magnetization transfer ratio with histopathologic correlation. J Comput Assist Tomogr 20:540-546
12. Dousset V, Armand JP, Lacoste D et al (1997) Magnetization transfer study of HIV encephalitis and progressive multifocal leukoencephalopathy. AJNR Am J Neuroradiol 18:859-901
13. Kasner SE, Galetta SL, McGowan JC, Grossman RI (1997) Magnetization transfer imaging in progressive multifocal leukoencephalopathy. Neurology 48:534-536
14. Silver NC, Barker GJ, MacManus DG et al (1996) Decreased magnetization transfer ratio due to demyelination: a case of central pontine myelinolysis. J Neurol Neurosurg Psychiatry 61:208-209
15. Thorpe JW, Barker GJ, Jones SJ et al (1995) Magnetisation transfer ratios and transverse magnetisation decay curves in optic neuritis: correlation with clinical findings and electrophysiology. J Neurol Neurosurg Psychiatry 59:487-492
16. Brochet B, Dousset V (1999) Pathological correlates of magnetization transfer imaging abnormalities in animal models and humans with multiple sclerosis. Neurology 53 (Suppl 3):S12-S17

17. Deloire-Grassin MSA, Brochet B, Quesson B et al (2000) In vivo evaluation of remyelination in rat brain by magnetization transfer imaging. J Neurol Sci 178:10-16
18. Kimura H, Grossman RI, Lenkinski RE, Gonzalez Scarano F (1996) Proton MR spectroscopy and magnetization transfer ratio in multiple sclerosis: correlative findings of active versus irreversible plaque disease. AJNR Am J Neuroradiol 17:1539-1547
19. Moffett JR, Namboodiri MAA, Cangro CB, Neale JH (1991) Immunohistochemical localization of N-acetylaspartate in rat brain. Neuroreport 2:131-134
20. Loevner LA, Grossman RI, McGowan JC et al (1995) Characterization of multiple sclerosis plaques with T_1-weighted MR and quantitative magnetization transfer. AJNR Am J Neuroradiol 16:1473-1479
21. Cercignani M, Iannucci G, Rocca MA et al (2000) Pathologic damage in MS assessed by diffusion-weighted and magnetization transfer MRI. Neurology 54:1139-1144
22. Inglese M, Rovaris M, Bianchi S et al (2001) Magnetic resonance imaging, magnetisation transfer imaging and diffusion weighted imaging correlates of optic nerve, brain and cervical cord damage in Leber's hereditary optic neuropathy. J Neurol Neurosurg Psychiatry 70:444-449
23. van Waesberghe JHTM, Kamphorst W, De Groot C et al (1999) Axonal loss in multiple sclerosis lesions: magnetic resonance imaging insights into substrates of disability. Ann Neurol 46:747-754
24. McGowan JC, McCormack TM, Grossman RI et al (1999) Diffuse axonal pathology detected with magnetization transfer imaging following brain injury in the pig. Magn Reson Med 41:727-733
25. Bagley LJ, Grossman RI, Galetta SL et al (1999) Characterization of white matter lesions in multiple sclerosis and traumatic brain injury as revealed by magnetization transfer contour plots. AJNR Am J Neuroradiol 20:977-981
26. van Buchem MA, McGowan JC, Kolson DL et al (1996) Quantitative volumetric magnetization transfer analysis in multiple sclerosis: estimation of macroscopic and microscopic disease burden. Magn Reson Med 36:632-636
27. Sormani MP, Iannucci G, Rocca MA et al (2000) Reproducibility of MTR histogram-derived measures of the brain on healthy volunteers. AJNR Am J Neuroradiol 21:133-136
28. Inglese M, Horsfield MA, Filippi M (2001) Scan-rescan variation of brain MTR histogram-derived measures from healthy volunteers using a semi-interleaved MT sequence. AJNR Am J Neuroradiol 22:681-684
29. Kermode AG, Tofts P, Thompson A et al (1990) Heterogeneity of blood-brain barrier changes in multiple sclerosis: an MRI study with gadolinium-DTPA enhancement. Neurology 40:229-235
30. Katz D, Taubenberger JK, Cannella B et al (1993) Correlation between magnetic resonance imaging findings and lesion development in multiple sclerosis. Ann Neurol 34:661-669
31. Filippi M, Rovaris M, Capra R et al (1998) A multi-center longitudinal study comparing the sensitivity of monthly MRI after standard and triple dose gadolinium-DTPA for monitoring disease activity in multiple sclerosis: implications for phase II clinical trials. Brain 121:2011-2020
32. Silver NC, Lai M, Symms MR et al (1998) Serial magnetization transfer imaging to characterize the early evolution of new MS lesions. Neurology 51:758-764
33. Campi A, Filippi M, Comi G et al (1996) Magnetization transfer ratios of contrast-enhancing and non-enhancing lesions in multiple sclerosis. Neuroradiology 38:115-119
34. Hiehle JF, Grossman RI, Ramer KN et al (1995) Magnetization transfer effects in MR-detected multiple sclerosis lesions: comparison with gadolinium-enhanced spin-echo images and non-enhanced T1-weighted images. AJNR Am J Neuroradiol 16:69-77
35. Petrella JR, Grossman RI, McGowan JC et al (1996) Multiple sclerosis lesions: relationship between MR enhancement pattern and magnetization transfer effect. AJNR Am J Neuroradiol 17:1041-1049

36. van Waesberghe JHTM, van Walderveen MAA, Castelijns JA et al (1998) Patterns of lesion development in multiple sclerosis: longitudinal observations with T1-weighted spin-echo and magnetization MR. AJNR Am J Neuroradiol 19:675-683
37. Filippi M, Rocca MA, Comi G (1998) Magnetization transfer ratios of multiple sclerosis lesions with variable durations of enhancement. J Neurol Sci 159:162-165
38. Filippi M, Rocca MA, Rizzo G et al (1998) Magnetization transfer ratios in MS lesions enhancing after different doses of gadolinium. Neurology 50:1289-1293
39. Filippi M, Rocca MA, Martino G et al (1998) Magnetization transfer changes in the normal appearing white matter precede the appearance of enhancing lesions in patients with multiple sclerosis. Ann Neurol 43:809-814
40. Goodkin DE, Rooney WD, Sloan R et al (1998) A serial study of new MS lesions and the white matter from which they arise. Neurology 51:1689-1697
41. Lai HM, Davie CA, Gass A et al (1997) Serial magnetization transfer ratios in gadolinium-enhancing lesions in multiple sclerosis. J Neurol 244:308-311
42. Filippi M, Comi G (1997) Magnetization transfer ratio changes in a symptomatic lesion of a patient at presentation with possible multiple sclerosis. J Neurol Sci 151:79-81
43. Dousset V, Gayou A, Brochet B, Caillé JM (1998) Early structural changes in acute MS lesions assessed by serial magnetization transfer studies. Neurology 51:1150-1155
44. Rocca MA, Mastronardo G, Rodegher M et al (1999) Long term changes of MT-derived measures from patients with relapsing-remitting and secondary-progressive multiple sclerosis. AJNR Am J Neuroradiol 20:821-827
45. Filippi M, Rocca MA, Sormani MP et al (1999) Short-term evolution of individual enhancing lesions studied with magnetization transfer imaging. Magn Reson Imaging 17:979-984
46. Kappos L, Moeri D, Radue EW et al (1999) Predictive value of gadolinium-enhanced MRI for relapse and changes in disability/impairment in multiple sclerosis: a met-analysis. Lancet 353:964-969
47. Filippi M, Campi A, Dousset V et al (1995) A magnetization transfer imaging study of normal-appearing white matter in multiple sclerosis. Neurology 45:478-482
48. Loevner LA, Grossman RI, Cohen JA et al (1995) Microscopic disease in normal-appearing white matter on conventional MR imaging in patients with multiple sclerosis: assessment with magnetization-transfer measurements. Radiology 96:511-515
49. Gass A, Barker GJ, Kidd D et al (1994) Correlation of magnetization transfer ratio with disability in multiple sclerosis. Ann Neurol 36:62-67
50. Guo AC, Jewells VL, Provenzale JM (2001) Analysis of normal-appearing white matter in multiple sclerosis: comparison of diffusion tensor MR imaging and magnetization transfer imaging. AJNR Am J Neuroradiol 22:1893-1900
51. Wong KT, Grossman RI, Boorstein JM et al (1995) Magnetization transfer imaging of perivascular hyperintense white matter in the elderly. AJNR Am J Neuroradiol 16:253-258
52. Rovaris M, Viti B, Ciboddo C et al (2000) Brain involvement in systemic immune-mediated diseases: a magnetic resonance and magnetization transfer imaging study. J Neurol Neurosurg Psychiatry 68:170-177
53. Gupta RK, Kathuria KM, Pradhan S (1999) Magnetization transfer MR imaging in CNS tuberculosis. AJNR Am J Neuroradiol 20:867-875
54. Rocca MA, Colombo B, Pratesi A et al (2000) A magnetization transfer imaging study of the brain in patients with migraine. Neurology 54:507-509
55. Tanabe JL, Ezekiel F, Jagust WJ et al (1999) Magnetization transfer ratio of white matter hyperintensities in subcortical ischemic vascular dementia. AJNR Am J Neuroradiol 20:839-844
56. Kato Y, Matsumura K, Kinosada Y et al (1997) Detection of pyramidal tract lesions in amyotrophic lateral sclerosis with magnetization-transfer measurements. AJNR Am J Neuroradiol 18:1541-1547
57. Iannucci G, Dichgans M, Rovaris M et al (2001) Correlations between clinical findings

and magnetization transfer imaging metrics of tissue damage in individuals with cerebral autosomal dominant arteriopathy with subcortical infarcts and leukoencephalopathy. Stroke 32:643-648

58. Inglese M, Salvi F, Iannucci G et al (2002) Magnetization transfer and diffusion tensor MR imaging of acute disseminated encephalomyelitis, AJNR Am J Neuroradiol 23:267-272

59. van Waesberghe JHTM, Castelijns JA, Scheltens P et al (1997) Comparison of four potential MR parameters for severe tissue destruction in multiple sclerosis lesions. Magn Reson Imaging 15:155-162

60. Rovaris M, Bozzali M, Rodegher M et al (1999) Brain MRI correlates of magnetization transfer imaging metrics in patients with multiple sclerosis. J Neurol Sci 166:58-63

61. Iannucci G, Rovaris M, Giacomotti L et al (2001) Correlations between measures of multiple sclerosis pathology derived from T2, T1, magnetization transfer and diffusion tensor MR imaging. AJNR Am J Neuroradiol 22:1462-1467

62. Pike GB, De Stefano N, Narayanan S et al (1999) Combined magnetization transfer and proton spectroscopic imaging in the assessment of pathologic brain lesions in multiple sclerosis. AJNR Am J Neuroradiol 20:829-837

63. Filippi M, Tortorella C, Rovaris M et al (2000) Changes in the normal appearing brain tissue and cognitive impairment in multiple sclerosis. J Neurol Neurosurg Psychiatry 68:157-161

64. Rovaris M, Bozzali M, Santuccio G et al (2001) In vivo assessment of the brain and cervical cord pathology of patients with primary progressive multiple sclerosis. Brain 124:2540-2549

65. Filippi M, Inglese M, Rovaris M et al (2000) Magnetization transfer imaging to monitor the evolution of MS: a one-year follow up study. Neurology 55:940-946

66. Iannucci G, Tortorella C, Rovaris M et al (2000) Prognostic value of MR and MTI findings at presentation in patients with clinically isolated syndromes suggestive of MS. AJNR Am J Neuroradiol 21:1034-1038

67. Filippi M, Iannucci G, Tortorella C et al (1999) Comparison of MS clinical phenotypes using conventional and magnetization transfer MRI. Neurology 52:588-594

68. Codella M, Rocca MA, Colombo B et al (2002) A preliminary study of magnetization transfer and diffusion tensor MRI of MS patients with fatigue. J Neurol 249:535-537

69. Rocca MA, Falini A, Colombo B et al (2002) Adaptive functional changes in the cerebral cortex of patients with non-disabling MS correlate with the extent of brain structural damage. Ann Neurol 51:330-339

70. Lee M, Reddy H, Johansen-Berg H et al (2000) The motor cortex shows adaptive functional changes to brain injury from multiple sclerosis. Ann Neurol 47:606-613

71. Reddy H, Narayanan S, Arnoutelis R et al (2000) Evidence for adaptive functional changes in the cerebral cortex with axonal injury from multiple sclerosis. Brain 123:2314-2320

72. Filippi M, Rocca MA, Falini A et al (2002) Correlations between structural CNS damage and functional MRI changes in primary progressive MS. NeuroImage 15:537-546

73. Adams CWM (1997) Pathology of multiple sclerosis: progression of the lesion. Br Med Bull 33:15-20

74. Allen IV, McKeown SR (1979) A histological, histochemical and biochemical study of the macroscopically normal white matter in multiple sclerosis. J Neurol Sci 41:81-89

75. Arstila AU, Riekkinen P, Rinne UK, Laitinen L (1973) Studies on the pathogenesis of multiple sclerosis. Participation of lysosomes on demyelination in the central nervous system white matter outside plaques. Eur Neurol 9:1-20

76. Bjartmar C, Kinkel RP, Kidd G et al (2001) Axonal loss in normal-appearing white matter in a patient with acute MS. Neurology 57:1248-1252

77. Evangelou N, Esiri MM, Smith S et al (2000) Quantitative pathological evidence for axonal loss in normal appearing white matter in multiple sclerosis. Ann Neurol 47:391-395

78. Pike GB, De Stefano N, Narayanan S et al (2000). Multiple sclerosis: magnetization transfer MR imaging of white matter before lesion appearance on T2-weighted images. Radiology 215:824-830
79. Filippi M, Rocca MA, Minicucci L et al (1999) Magnetization transfer imaging of patients with definite MS and negative conventional MRI. Neurology 52:845-848
80. Santos AC, Narayanan S, De Stefano N et al (2002) Magnetization transfer can predict clinical evolution in patients with multiple sclerosis. J Neurol 249:662-668
81. Tortorella C, Viti B, Bozzali M et al (2000) A magnetization transfer histogram study of normal appearing brain tissue in multiple sclerosis. Neurology 54:186-193
82. Brex PA, Leary SM, Plant GT et al (2001) Magnetization transfer imaging in patients with clinically isolated syndromes suggestive of multiple sclerosis. AJNR Am J Neuroradiol 22:947-951
83. Kaiser JS, Grossman RI, Polansky M et al (2000) Magnetization transfer histogram analysis of monosymptomatic episodes of neurologic dysfunction: preliminary findings. AJNR Am J Neuroradiol 21:1043-1047
84. Siger-Zajdel M, Filippi M, Selmaj K (2002) MTR discloses subtle changes in the normal-appearing tissue from relatives of patients with MS. Neurology 58:317-320
85. Cercignani M, Bozzali M, Iannucci G et al (2001) Magnetisation transfer ratio and mean diffusivity of normal-appearing white and gray matter from patients with multiple sclerosis. J Neurol Neurosurg Psychiatry 70:311-317
86. Filippi M, Rocca MA, Moiola L et al (1999) MRI and MTI changes in the brain and cervical cord from patients with Devic's neuromyelitis optica. Neurology 53:1705-1710
87. Ge Y, Grossman RI, Udupa JK et al (2002) Magnetization transfer ratio histogram analysis of normal-appearing gray matter and normal-appearing white matter in multiple sclerosis. J Comput Assist Tomogr 26:62-68
88. Kidd D, Barkhof F, McConnel R et al (1999) Cortical lesions in multiple sclerosis. Brain 122:17-26
89. Peterson JW, Bo L, Mork S et al (2001) Transected neurites, apoptotic neurons, and reduced inflammation in cortical multiple sclerosis lesions. Ann Neurol 50:389-400
90. Ge Y, Grossman RI, Udupa JK et al (2001) Magnetization transfer ratio histogram analysis of gray matter in relapsing-remitting multiple sclerosis. AJNR Am J Neuroradiol 22:470-475
91. Rovaris M, Filippi M, Minicucci L et al (2000) Cortical/subcortical disease burden and cognitive impairment in multiple sclerosis. AJNR Am J Neuroradiol 21:402-408
92. Filippi M, Bozzali M, Comi G (2001) Magnetization transfer and diffusion tensor MR imaging of basal ganglia from patients with multiple sclerosis. J Neurol Sci 183:69-72
93. Codella M, Rocca MA, Colombo B et al (2002) Cerebral gray matter pathology and fatigue in patients with multiple sclerosis: a preliminary study. J Neurol Sci 194:71-74
94. Rudick RA, Fisher E, Lee JC et al (1999) Use of the brain parenchymal fraction to measure whole brain atrophy in relapsing-remitting MS. Neurology 53:1698-1704
95. Filippi M, Rovaris M, Iannucci G et al (2000) Whole brain volume changes in progressive MS patients treated with cladribine. Neurology 55:1714-1718
96. Dehmeshki J, Ruto AC, Arridge S et al (2001) Analysis of MTR histograms in multiple sclerosis using principal components and multiple discriminant analysis. Magn Reson Med 46:600-609
97. Kalkers NF, Hintzen RQ, van Waesberghe JH et al (2001) Magnetization transfer histogram parameters reflect all dimensions of MS pathology, including atrophy. J Neurol Sci 184:155-162
98. Rovaris M, Holtmannspötter M, Rocca MA et al (2002) The contribution of cervical cord MRI and brain magnetization transfer imaging to the assessment of individual patients with multiple sclerosis: a preliminary study. Mult Scler 8:52-58
99. van Buchem MA, Grossman RI, Armstrong C et al (1998) Correlation of volumetric magnetization transfer imaging with clinical data in MS. Neurology 50:1609-1617
100. Iannucci G, Minicucci L, Rodegher ME et al (1999) Correlations between clinical and

MRI involvement in multiple sclerosis: assessment using T1, T2 and MT histograms. J Neurol Sci 171:121-129

101. Dehmeshki J, Barker GJ, Tofts PS (2002) Classification of disease subgroup and correlation with disease severity using magnetic resonance imaging whole-brain histograms: application to magnetization transfer ratios and multiple sclerosis. IEEE Trans Med Imaging 21:320-331

102. Rovaris M, Filippi M, Falautano M et al (1998) Relation between MR abnormalities and patterns of cognitive impairment in multiple sclerosis. Neurology 50:1601-1608

103. Comi G, Rovaris M, Falautano M et al (1999) A multiparametric MRI study of frontal lobe dementia in multiple sclerosis. J Neurol Sci 171:135-144

104. Phillips MD, Grossman RI, Miki Y et al (1998) Comparison of T2 lesion volume and magnetization transfer ratio histogram analysis and of atrophy and measures of lesion burden in patients with multiple sclerosis. AJNR Am J Neuroradiol 19:1055-1060

105. Bozzali M, Rocca MA, Iannucci G et al (1999) Magnetization transfer histogram analysis of the cervical cord in patients wth multiple sclerosis. AJNR Am J Neuroradiol 20:1803-1808

106. Boorstein JM, Moonis G, Boorstein SM et al (1997) Optic neuritis: imaging with magnetization transfer. AJNR Am J Neuroradiol 169:1709-1712

107. Silver NC, Barker CJ, Losseff NA et al (1997) Magnetization transfer ratio measurements in the cervical spinal cord: a preliminary study in multiple sclerosis. Neuroradiology 39:441-445

108. Lycklama à Nijeholt GJ, Castelijns JA, Lazeron RH et al (2000) Magnetization transfer ratio of the spinal cord in multiple sclerosis: relationship to atrophy and neurologic disability. J Neuroimaging 10:67-72

109. Filippi M, Bozzali M, Horsfield MA et al (2000) A conventional and magnetization transfer MRI study of the cervical cord in patients with multiple sclerosis. Neurology 54:207-213

110. Rovaris M, Bozzali M, Santuccio G et al (2000) Relative contributions of brain and cervical cord pathology to MS disability: a study with MTR histogram analysis. J Neurol Neurosurg Psychiatry 69:723-727

111. Rocca MA, Filippi M, Herzog J et al (2001) A magnetic resonance imaging study of the cervical cord of patients with CADASIL. Neurology 56:1392-1394

112. Inglese M, Ghezzi A, Bianchi S et al (2002) MS irreversible disability and tissue loss: a conventional and MT MRI study of the optic nerves. Arch Neurol 59:250-255

113. Filippi M, Dousset V, McFarland HF et al (2002) The role of MRI in the diagnosis and monitoring of multiple sclerosis. Consensus report of the "White Matter Study Group" of the International Society for Magnetic Resonance in Medicine. J Magn Reson Imaging 15:499-504

114. Richert ND, Ostuni JL, Bash CN et al (1998) Serial whole-brain magnetization transfer imaging in patients with relapsing-remitting multiple sclerosis at baseline and during treatment with interferon beta-1b. AJNR Am J Neuroradiol 19:1705-1713

115. Richert ND, Ostuni JL, Bash CN et al (2001) Interferon beta-1b and intravenous methylprednisolone promote lesion recovery in multiple sclerosis. Mult Scler 7:49-58

116. Kita M, Goodkin DE, Bacchetti P et al (2000) Magnetization transfer ratio in new MS lesions before and during therapy with IFNß-1a. Neurology 54:1741-1745

117. Filippi M, Inglese M, van Waesberghe JH et al (2002) The effect of interferon beta-1b on quantities derived from MT MRI in secondary progressive multiple sclerosis (abstract). J Neurol 249 (Suppl 1):I/168

118. Filippi M, Iannucci G, Sormani MP et al (2002) The effect of intravenous immunoglobulins on quantities derived from MT MRI in secondary progressive multiple sclerosis (abstract). J Neurol 249 (Suppl 1):I/115-116

119. Sled JG, Pike GB (2001) Quantitative imaging of magnetization transfer exchange and relaxation properties in vivo using MRI. Magn Reson Med 46:923-931

120. Ropele S, Strasser-Fuchs S, Seifert T et al (2002) Development of active multiple sclerosis lesions: a quantitative MT study (abstract). Proc Intl Soc Magn Reson Med 10:180
121. Sled JG, Levesque I, Narayanan S et al (2002) The role of edema and demyelination in T1 black holes: a quantitative magnetization transfer study (abstract). Proc Intl Soc Mag Reson Med 10:181
122. Dehmeshki J, Silver NC, Leary S et al (2001). Magnetisation transfer ratio histogram analysis of primary progressive and other multiple sclerosis subgroups. J Neurol Sci 185:11-17
123. Dehmeshki J, Chard DT, Leary S et al (2002). Magnetisation transfer histograms in primary progressive multiple sclerosis: grey matter changes relate to disability and principal component analysis shows this most sensitively (abstract). Proc Intl Soc Mag Reson Med 10:179

Chapter 3

Diffusion-Weighted MRI

M. FILIPPI, M.A. ROCCA

Introduction

Although conventional T2-weighted magnetic resonance imaging (MRI) is sensitive for the detection of multiple sclerosis (MS) lesions, it is not without important limitations. First, MRI lacks specificity with regard to the heterogeneous pathological substrates of individual lesions, and in consequence does not allow tissue damage to be quantified. Edema, inflammation, demyelination, remyelination, gliosis, and axonal loss [1] all have a similar appearance of hyperintensity on T2-weighted images. Secondly, T2-weighted images do not delineate tissue damage occurring in the normal-appearing white (NAWM) and gray matter (NAGM), which usually represents a large portion of the brain tissue from MS patients and is known to be damaged in MS [2-5]. These limitations are only partially overcome by the use of postcontrast T1-weighted scans. Gadolinium-enhanced T1-weighted images allow active and inactive lesions to be distinguished from each other [6, 7], since enhancement occurs as a result of increased blood-brain barrier (BBB) permeability [8] and corresponds to areas with ongoing inflammation [9]. However, the activity of the lesions as demonstrated on postcontrast T1-weighted imaging still does not provide information on tissue damage. Hypointense lesions on T1-weighted images correspond to areas where chronic severe tissue disruption has occurred [10], and their extent correlates with the clinical severity of the disease and its evolution over time [11, 12]. Still, the extent of T1-hypointense lesions may not correspond to the severity of the intrinsic lesion pathology and provides no information about NAWM and NAGM damage. Recently, several other MRI techniques, including diffusion-weighted (DW) MRI, have been used extensively to improve our understanding of the evolution of MS.

Diffusion is the microscopic random translational motion of molecules in a fluid system. In the central nervous system (CNS), diffusion is influenced by the microstructural components of tissue, including cell membranes and organelles. The diffusion coefficient of biological tissues (which can be measured in vivo by MRI) is therefore lower than the diffusion coefficient in free water and for this reason is named "apparent diffusion coefficient" (ADC) [13]. Pathological processes which modify tissue integrity, resulting in a loss or increased permeability of "restricting" barriers, can lead to an increase of the ADC. Since some cellular structures are aligned on the scale of an image pixel, the measurement of diffusion is also dependent on the direction in which diffusion is measured. As a consequence, diffusion measurements can give information about the size, shape, integrity, and orientation of tissues [14]. A measure of diffusion that is independent of the orientation of structures is provided by the mean diffusivity ($\bar{D}$), the average of the ADCs measured in three orthogonal directions. A full characterization of diffusion can be obtained in terms of a tensor [15], a 3 × 3 matrix which accounts for the correlation existing between molecular displacement along orthogonal directions. From the tensor, it is possible to derive $\bar{D}$, equal to one-third of its trace, and some other dimensionless indices of anisotropy. One of the most used of these indices is named "fractional anisotropy" (FA) [16, 17].

The pathological elements of MS have the potential to alter the permeability or geometry of structural barriers to water molecular diffusion in the brain. The present review outlines the major contributions of DW-MRI to the quantification of MS-related damage and to the understanding of MS pathophysiology.

Normal-Appearing White Matter

All studies of water diffusion in MS have shown consistently that ADC or $\bar{D}$ values of NAWM are higher than those of corresponding white matter from controls, but lower than those measured in T2-visible lesions [18-32]. DTI studies also showed that FA values of NAWM are lower than those of corresponding white matter from controls and higher than those of T2-visible lesions [22, 23, 27, 30-32]. All these studies are consistent with the findings of other pathological quantitative MRI studies showing that tissue damage does occur outside T2-visible lesions [2]. Although these results indicate a net loss and disorganization of structural barriers to water molecular motion in the NAWM, the possible pathological substrates of these findings have not yet been defined. Subtle changes are known to occur in the NAWM from patients with MS, including diffuse astrocytic hyperplasia, patchy edema, perivascular infiltration, gliosis, abnormally thin myelin and axonal loss [33]. While all these processes might reduce FA, myelin and axonal loss should lead to increased water diffusivity. As a consequence, they are the most likely contributors to the increased water diffusivity and decreased FA observed in the NAWM.

Several studies assessed DW-MRI changes in different brain regions and showed that NAWM changes in MS are widespread, but tend to be more severe in sites where macroscopic MS lesions are usually located [23, 27, 30, 31] and in periplaque regions [34, 35]. Intriguingly, significant DW-MRI changes have been shown in the internal capsule and corpus callosum of patients with primary progressive MS [30], which might at least partially explain the locomotor disability and cognitive impairment seen in these patients [36]. That NAWM damage is widespread in MS has also been shown in a recent study, where $\bar{D}$ was measured in a large portion of brain NAWM [31].

DW-MRI changes in the NAWM have been reported to correlate moderately with the extent of macroscopic lesions seen on conventional MR images [23, 24, 30, 31, 37, 38]. This suggests that these subtle NAWM changes are not merely the result of wallerian degeneration of axons traversing larger lesions, but may also represent small focal abnormalities beyond the resolution of conventional scanning and independent of larger lesions.

As previously shown using magnetization transfer imaging [39, 40], two studies detected increased $\bar{D}$ values in NAWM areas subsequently involved by new MS lesions [25, 26], suggesting that focal edema and demyelination beyond the resolution of conventional MRI may play a part in the NAWM changes preceding new lesion formation in MS.

Normal-Appearing Gray Matter

In normal brain, gray matter and white matter have different diffusion characteristics. In gray matter, diffusion is isotropic when averaged on a voxel scale, while it is extremely anisotropic in white matter due to the directionality of the myelin fiber tracts [41]. Using a segmentation technique based on FA thresholds and histogram analysis, Cercignani et al. [31] showed that $\bar{D}$ of brain NAGM from MS patients is higher than that of brain NAGM from sex- and age-matched healthy volunteers. This indicates that brain GM is not spared by the MS pathological process. Previous postmortem studies [3-5] showed that lesions are relatively frequent in the cerebral GM of patients with MS. As a consequence, one explanation of this finding might be the presence of a certain number of discrete MS lesions in the NAGM of MS patients that go undetected on conventional T2-weighted imaging because they are usually small [3], have relaxation characteristics which result in poor contrast against and normal GM, and, in the case of cortical lesions, because of partial volume effects with surrounding cerebrospinal fluid. An alternative explanation (not necessarily exclusive of the first) of the $\bar{D}$ changes in NAGM might be retrograde degeneration of GM neurons secondary to the damage of fibers traversing MS white matter lesions. The supposition hat retrograde degeneration may have a role in explaining NAGM changes in MS is supported by the correlations found between T2-visible lesion volume and NAGM $\bar{D}$ [31, 38]. The presence of NAGM damage in MS fits well with the frequent demonstration of cognitive impairment in patients with MS [42]. Rovaris et al. [43] found a moderate correlation between a cognitive impairment index and $\bar{D}$ of the NAGM in 34 mildly disabled relapsing-remitting MS patients. Using DW-MRI, Bozzali et al. [44] have recently demonstrated that NAGM changes are more pronounced in patients with secondary progressive and primary progressive MS than in patients with the relapsing-remitting course of the disease, whereas Rovaris et al. [45] showed that NAWM and NAGM pathology is more severe in patients with secondary progressive MS than in patients with primary progressive MS. These findings suggest that NAGM pathological abnormalities might yet be an additional factor contributing to the worsening of clinical disability in patients with progressive MS.

DW-MRI has also been used to investigate whether subtle structural changes can be detected in the basal ganglia of patients with MS [46]. In a study of 31 patients with MS, no DW-MRI changes were found in any of the basal ganglia regions studied. This confirms that basal ganglia damage is modest in MS and suggests that the positron emission tomography [47] and functional MRI [48] changes detected in the basal ganglia of MS patients are more likely to be secondary to diaschisis phenomena than to intrinsic structural changes.

Lesions Visible on Conventional MR Images

All studies of water diffusion have shown highly variable ADC, $\bar{D}$, and FA values in macroscopic MS lesions [18-31]. This is consistent with the known pathological heterogeneity of MS lesions [49, 50]. Nevertheless, water diffusion abnormalities are, on average, different in different types of MS lesions. All investigators have shown higher ADC or $\bar{D}$ values in nonenhancing T1-hypointense than in nonenhancing T1-isointense lesions [21-23, 27-30]. T1-hypointense lesions are those where severe tissue loss has occurred [10, 51] and their extent correlates with disease progression in patients with secondary progressive MS [11]. Although postmortem studies correlating histopathology and DW-MRI changes are needed, this observation shows the potential for DW-MRI to provide quantitative metrics for monitoring tissue damage in MS. Conflicting results have been achieved in comparisons of ADC or $\bar{D}$ in enhancing versus nonenhancing lesions. Some studies reported higher ADC or $\bar{D}$ values in nonenhancing than in enhancing lesions [21, 22, 29], but others, based on larger samples of patients and lesions, did not report any significant difference between the two kinds of lesions [23, 27, 30]. This discrepancy confirms that variable degrees of tissue damage occur in new enhancing lesions in MS [51-54] and might reflect different lesion ages ($\bar{D}$ increases sharply at the time of enhancement onset and then decreases rapidly in the next few weeks [25, 26]). On the other hand, FA has always been found to be lower in enhancing than in nonenhancing lesions [22, 30]. Future longitudinal studies are warranted to address the important question of how much of this tissue disorganization in enhancing lesions is permanent (i.e., related to axonal loss) and how much is transient (i.e., related to edema, demyelination, and remyelination).

Several studies have shown that water diffusivity is markedly increased in ring-enhancing lesions compared to homogeneously enhancing lesions [27-29], or in the nonenhancing portions of enhancing lesions compared with enhancing portions [28]. Markedly reduced FA values have also been found in ring-enhancing lesions [27]. All of this again suggests that pronounced tissue destruction can occur in active MS lesions.

The above findings on the one hand confirm the pathological heterogeneity of MS lesions, and on the other they show that measures derived from conventional MR images (extent of T2-visible lesions, presence of enhancement, extent of "black holes") are not able to fully describe this heterogeneity. They also indicate that quantities derived from DW-MRI have the potential to improve dramatically our ability to define and monitor the mechanisms underlying MS tissue damage and repair, since the various pathological substrates of the disease (edema, inflammation, demyelination, remyelination, reactive gliosis, and axonal loss) are likely to have differing impacts on the size, shape, integrity, and orientation of water-filled spaces.

$\bar{D}$ and FA of MS lesions were found to correlate strongly with lesion extent on T2- and T1-weighted images [30]. This provides support for the concept that, on average, the size of lesions and the severity of the tissue damage within them run in parallel. A significant correlation between $\bar{D}$ and FA of macroscopic MS lesions has also been reported [22, 30]. This correlation was, however, far from being a strict relationship. Since tissue damage alone would both increase $\bar{D}$ and decrease FA, this observation suggests the potential of serial DW-MRI scans to monitor tissue repair. For example, marked glial proliferation would decrease both $\bar{D}$ and FA in concert, thus reducing the magnitude of the correlation that would result from a marked preponderance of tissue damage over tissue repair.

Aggregate of Different Brain Tissues

As shown for magnetization transfer imaging [55-58], DW-MRI changes can be assessed using histogram analysis, thus obtaining quantities reflecting together the macro- and microscopic MS lesion burden in aggregates of different brain tissues. Cercignani et al. [24] measured $\bar{D}$ in a large portion of the central brain from 35 patients with mildly disabling relapsing-remitting MS and compared it with that of 24 age- and sex-matched healthy volunteers. Significantly higher brain $\bar{D}$ and lower histogram peak height were found in patients. Similar results were found by two other studies [37, 59]. In the study by Cercignani et al. [24], magnetization transfer ratio (MTR) histograms were also produced and no correlation was found between average MTR and $\bar{D}$ taken from the histograms. The lack of correlation between MTR and $\bar{D}$ in the brain tissue is likely to be the result of the complex relationship between destructive (inflammation, demyelination, and axonal loss) and reparative (remyelination and gliosis) mechanisms and their variable effects on MTR and $\bar{D}$ values. Using histogram analysis, Cercignani et al. [37] also showed significant changes of FA histogram-derived metrics in a large cohort of MS patients with various disease phenotypes. This study also showed a moderate correlation between brain $\bar{D}$ and FA, as previously described for T2-visible lesions [22, 30].

All the above results are affected by the presence of macroscopic MS lesions and subtle changes in NAWM and NAGM. More recent studies have assessed water diffusivity changes in normal-appearing brain tissue (NABT) by excluding from the histogram analysis those pixels belonging to T2-visible lesions [38, 43, 60, 61]. Increased water diffusivity was found in the NABT of patients with MS [61] and in patients with Leber's hereditary optic neuropathy [60] compared to controls. Interestingly, patients with MS also had higher NABT $\bar{D}$ than those with acute disseminated encephalomyelitis [61]. No significant correlation was found between magnetization transfer and DW-MRI-derived metrics of the NABT [38], confirming previous results assessing the correlation between these quantities taken from histograms of brain tissue containing T2-visible lesions [24].

Clearly, using histogram analysis, information related to the status of specific brain structures is inevitably lost. However, in the context of MS clinical trials, it may be unfeasible to measure $\bar{D}$ and FA changes from several different brain regions and tissues, whereas a quantitative measure reflecting overall lesion burden might be a desirable outcome measure.

Correlations with MS Clinical Manifestations, Functional MRI Activations, and Disability

Significant correlations between DW-MRI findings and clinical manifestations of MS or disability were not found in some of the earliest studies [20, 21, 23, 24], perhaps because of the relatively small samples studied [20], the limited brain coverage [20, 21], or the narrow range of disabilities that was considered [23, 24]. With improved DW-MRI technology and increased numbers of patients studied, correlations between DW-MRI findings and MS clinical manifestations or disability are now emerging [30, 37, 43, 59, 62].

Average lesion $\bar{D}$, but not average lesion FA, was found to be significantly correlated, albeit moderately, with clinical disability in a study of 78 patients with MS [30]. The lack of correlation between disability and FA indicates that the loss of overall impediment to diffusional motion is more important than the loss of tissue anisotropy in determining patients' clinical status. This fits well with the concept that loss of anisotropy might also result from reparative mechanisms. Interestingly, in patients with secondary progressive MS a moderate and significant correlation was found between average lesion $\bar{D}$ or FA and disability, whereas no significant correlation was found between disability and T2-visible lesion volume. On the contrary, a significant correlation between disability and T2 lesion volume was found in patients with relapsing-remitting MS, where, in turn, there was no correlation between average lesion $\bar{D}$ or FA and disability. These findings suggest that mechanisms leading to disability are likely to be different in patients with relapsing-remitting and those with secondary progressive MS. Although caution must be exercised, one might speculate that new lesion formation is a relevant pathological aspect in relapsing-remitting MS, whereas tissue loss in pre-existing lesions is one of the pathological hallmarks of secondary progressive MS. As a consequence, these results indicate DW-MRI measures as promising MR markers to be used in addition to conventional MRI to monitor the evolution of secondary progressive MS. Consistent with these observations, it has been shown that water diffusivity in the whole of the brain tissue [59] and in T2-visible lesions [62] is significantly increased in patients with secondary progressive MS compared to those with relapsing-remitting MS. Castriota Scanderbeg et al. [62] also found strong correlations between average lesion diffusivity, disability, and disease duration. Cercignani et al. [37] found a strong correlation between disability and FA histogram peak position in patients with secondary progressive MS. Finally, a recent multiparametric MR study has shown that a composite MR score, based on the T1-hypointense lesion volume, brain N-acetylaspartate to creatine ratio, and brain $\bar{D}$, is strictly correlated with the level of MS-related disability [63].

Rovaris et al. [43] correlated DW-MRI findings with cognitive impairment in 34 patients with relapsing-remitting MS. They found moderate correlations between several DW-MRI quantities and neuropsychological test scores, whereas no correlation was found between any of the DW-MRI quantities and physical disability.

More recently, in patients with relapsing-remitting [64] and primary progressive MS [65, 66], moderate to strong correlations have also been found between the severity of structural changes of the NABT (as measured using magnetization transfer and DW-MRI) and the relative activations of several cortical areas located in a widespread network for sensorimotor and multimodal integration, measured using functional MRI. This suggests that not only macroscopic MS lesions, but also subtle NABT changes can cause adaptive cortical reorganization with the potential to limit the functional consequences of MS-related structural damage.

Diffusion Tensor MRI Tractography

DW-MRI provides a method by which it may become possible to obtain in vivo human connectivity data both rapidly and noninvasively. Due to the different tissue anisotropies, DW-MRI is able not only to distinguish white matter from gray matter, but also to elucidate the macroscopic volume-averaged orientation of the microstructure therein. The anisotropy provides the basis of diffusion tensor (DT) tractography methods, developed to determine the pathways of anatomical CNS connections through the white matter in vivo. There are several methodological limitations to DT-MRI that degrade the information about the spatial orientation of fiber tracts contained within the DT. These include the poor resolution of DW-MRI data in comparison with the size of fiber tracts and the low signal-to-noise ratio of the DW-MRI data from which the DT is estimated, which introduces errors in the directional information derived from it.

Recently, several authors have developed different tractography techniques that utilize the directional and anisotropy information contained in a given voxel to connect neighboring voxels and to visualize white matter tracts in vivo (67-69) (Fig. 1). The development of these methods to identify and segment a single brain tract is important because this would allow a detailed assessment of damage within it, and a subsequent comparison with relevant clinical data. Tench and coworkers [70] used this technique to map the corpus callosum and the pyramidal tracts from 14 MS patients and 10 controls and to measure the corresponding ADC values within these tracts. The ADC was significantly higher in patients than in controls, and it was higher in the corpus callosum than in the pyramidal tracts in both groups. The application of such methods to segment the different function-

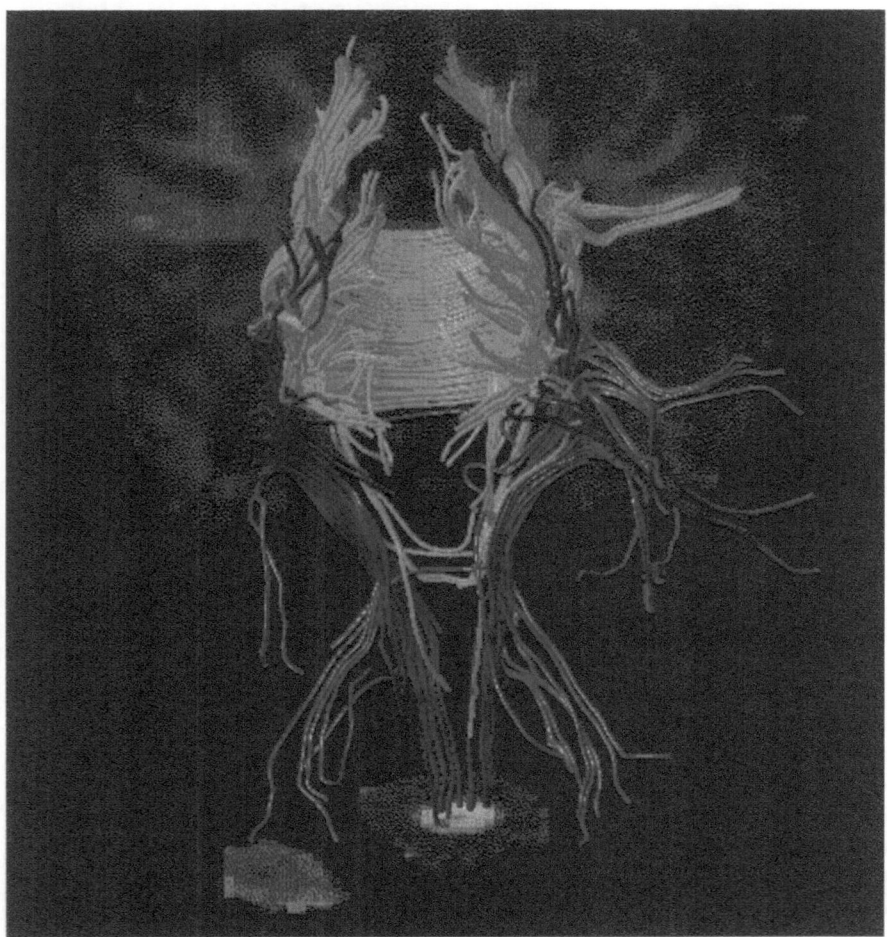

Fig. 1. 3D projection of diffusion tracking of corpus callosum fibers (*green*) and of the pyramidal tracts (*red*). (Courtesy of Dr. Derek Jones, Section of Old Age Psychiatry, Maudsley Hospital, Denmark Hill, London)

al white matter structures in MS patients might allow the strength of the correlations between clinical and MRI findings to be improved.

Optic Nerve and Spinal Cord

Although DW-MRI of the optic nerve and the spinal cord would be desirable to achieve a more complete picture of how MS causes irreversible disability, DW-MRI in these brain regions presents considerable technical challenges.

Nevertheless, successful DW-MRI of the optic nerve [71, 72] and spinal cord [73-78] has been recently carried out in normal controls and patients with different neurological conditions. At present, only one study assessed water diffusion in seven cord lesions of three MS patients with locomotor disability [73]. They found that MS cord lesions had increased $\bar{D}$ compared to cord tissue from healthy volunteers. Another study assessed water diffusion in the optic nerve of patients with optic neuritis [71], demonstrating significantly different optic nerve ADC values between controls and patients. This study also showed that ADC differs between acute and chronic optic neuritis cases: ADC was found to be decreased in the acute (inflammatory) stage of optic neuritis, and increased in the chronic phase.

With the progressive advance of DW-MRI technology, it is likely that measurements of water diffusion characteristics in the spinal cord (Fig. 2) and optic nerve of patients with MS will increasingly be obtained. Hopefully, this should lead to a more accurate assessment of MS pathology in vivo, and, as a consequence, to a better understanding of the pathophysiology of this disease.

Conclusions

Conventional MRI is limited by its lack of specificity for the heterogeneous pathological substrates of MS lesions and by its inaccuracy in measuring the overall lesion burden of MS. DW-MRI is one of the most promising new MR techniques for overcoming these limitations, at least partially. It allows the amount of tissue damage in MS lesions to be quantified, and makes it possible to detect more subtle changes occurring in NAWM and NAGM. Although DW-MRI changes reflect a net loss of structural organization, we can only speculate on the possible pathological substrates of such changes. Investigation of the relationship between DW-MRI metrics and other MR quantities derived from magnetization transfer imaging, MR spectroscopy, and functional MRI might increase our understanding of

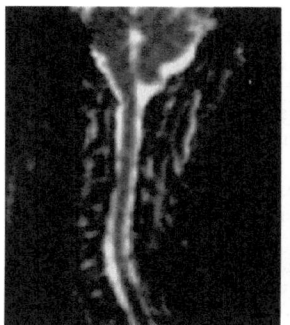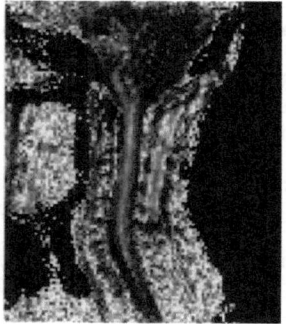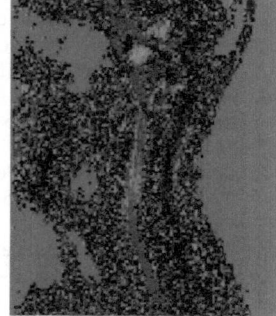

Fig. 2. Sagittal diffusion tensor MRI of the cervical cord, collected using a SENSE single-shot EPI pulse sequence: a) mean diffusivity map; b) fractional anisotropy map (lattice index); c) map of directionality (*blue* represents the vertical direction)

this important issue. Postmortem studies correlating DW-MRI findings with the histopathology of MS are also warranted, as well as longitudinal studies of patients with various MS phenotypes to elucidate the correlation between evolving diffusion abnormalities and the development of irreversible disability.

References

1. McDonald WI, Miller DH, Barnes D (1992) The pathological evolution of multiple sclerosis. Neuropathol Appl Neurobiol 18:319-334
2. Filippi M, Tortorella C, Bozzali M (1999) Normal-appearing-white-matter changes in multiple sclerosis: the contribution of magnetic resonance techniques. Mult Scler 5:273-282
3. Kidd D, Barkhof F, McConnel R et al (1999) Cortical lesions in multiple sclerosis. Brain 122:17-26
4. Brownell B, Hughes JT (1962) The distribution of plaques in the cerebrum in multiple sclerosis. J Neurol Neurosurg Psychiatry 25:315-320
5. Lumsden CE (1970) The neuropathology of multiple sclerosis. In: Vinken PJ, Bruyn GW eds. Handbook of clinical neurology, vol 9. North-Holland, Amsterdam, pp 217-309
6. McFarland HF, Frank JA, Albert PS et al (1992) Using gadolinium-enhanced magnetic resonance imaging to monitor disease activity in multiple sclerosis. Ann Neurol 32:758-766
7. Miller DH, Barkhof F, Nauta JJP (1993) Gadolinium enhancement increased the sensitivity of MRI in detecting disease activity in MS. Brain 116:1077-1094
8. Kermode AG, Tofts P, Thompson AJ et al (1990) Heterogeneity of blood-brain barrier changes in multiple sclerosis: an MRI study with gadolinium-DTPA enhancement. Neurology 40:229-235
9. Katz D, Taubenberger JK, Cannella B et al (1993) Correlation between magnetic resonance imaging findings and lesion development in multiple sclerosis. Ann Neurol 34:661-669
10. van Walderveen MAA, Kamphorst W, Scheltens P et al (1998) Histopathologic correlate of hypointense lesions on T1-weighted spin-echo MRI in multiple sclerosis. Neurology 50:1282-1288
11. Truyen L, van Waesberghe JHTM, van Walderveen MAA et al (1996) Accumulation of hypointense lesions ("black holes") on T1 spin-echo MRI correlates with disease progression in multiple sclerosis. Neurology 47:1469-1476
12. Rovaris M, Comi G, Rocca MA et al (1999) Relevance of hypointense lesions on fast fluid-attenuated inversion recovery MR images as a marker of disease severity in cases of multiple sclerosis. AJNR Am J Neuroradiol 20:813-820
13. Le Bihan D, Breton E, Lallemand D et al (1986) MR imaging of intravoxel incoherent motions: application to diffusion and perfusion in neurologic disorders. Radiology 161:401-407
14. Le Bihan D, Turner R, Pekar J, Moonen CTW (1991) Diffusion and perfusion imaging by gradient sensitization: design, strategy and significance. J Magn Reson Imaging 1:7-8
15. Basser PJ, Mattiello J, Le Bihan D (1994) Estimation of the effective self-diffusion tensor from the NMR spin-echo. J Magn Reson B 103:247-254
16. Pierpaoli C, Jezzard P, Basser PJ et al (1996) Diffusion tensor MR imaging of the human brain. Radiology 201:637-648
17. Basser PJ, Pierpaoli C (1996) Microstructural features measured using diffusion tensor imaging. J Magn Reson B 111:209-219
18. Larsson HBW, Thomsen C, Frederiksen J et al (1992) In vivo magnetic resonance dif-

fusion measurement in the brain of patients with multiple sclerosis. Magn Reson Imaging 10:7-12

19. Christiansen P, Gideon P, Thomsen C et al (1993) Increased water self-diffusion in chronic plaques and in apparently normal white matter in patients with multiple sclerosis. Acta Neurol Scand 87:195-199

20. Horsfield MA, Lai M, Webb SL et al (1996) Apparent diffusion coefficients in benign and secondary progressive multiple sclerosis by nuclear magnetic resonance. Magn Reson Med 36:393-400

21. Droogan AG, Clark CA, Werring DJ et al (1999) Comparison of multiple sclerosis clinical subgroups using navigated spin echo diffusion-weighted imaging. Magn Reson Imaging 17:653-661

22. Werring DJ, Clark CA, Barker GJ et al (1999) Diffusion tensor imaging of lesions and normal-appearing white matter in multiple sclerosis. Neurology 52:1626-1632

23. Filippi M, Iannucci G, Cercignani M et al (2000) A quantitative study of water diffusion in multiple sclerosis lesions and normal-appearing white matter using echo-planar imaging. Arch Neurol 57:1017-1021

24. Cercignani M, Iannucci G, Rocca MA et al (2000) Pathologic damage in MS assessed by diffusion-weighted and magnetization transfer MRI. Neurology 54:1139-1144

25. Rocca MA, Cercignani M, Iannucci G et al (2000) Weekly diffusion-weighted imaging of normal-appearing white matter in MS. Neurology 55:882-884

26. Werring DJ, Brassat D, Droogan AG et al (2000) The pathogenesis of lesions and normal-appearing white matter changes in multiple sclerosis. A serial diffusion MRI study. Brain 123:1667-1676

27. Bammer R, Augustin M, Strasser-Fuchs S et al (2000) Magnetic resonance diffusion tensor imaging for characterizing diffuse and focal white matter abnormalities in multiple sclerosis. Magn Reson Med 44:583-59

28. Nusbaum AO, Lu D, Tang CY, Atlas SW (2000) Quantitative diffusion measurements in focal multiple sclerosis lesions: correlations with appearance on T1-weighted MR images. AJR Am J Roentgenol 175:821-825

29. Roychowdhury S, Maldijan JA, Grossman RI (2000) Multiple sclerosis: comparison of trace apparent diffusion coefficients with MR enhancement pattern of lesions. AJNR Am J Neuroradiol 21:869-874

30. Filippi M, Cercignani M, Inglese M et al (2001) Diffusion tensor magnetic resonance imaging in multiple sclerosis. Neurology 56:304-311

31. Cercignani M, Bozzali M, Iannucci G et al (2001) Magnetisation transfer ratio and mean diffusivity of normal appearing white and grey matter from patients with multiple sclerosis. J Neurol Neurosurg Psychiatry 70:311-317

32. Ciccarelli O, Werring DJ, Wheeler-Kingshott CA et al (2001) Investigation of MS normal-appearing brain using diffusion tensor MRI with clinical correlations. Neurology 56:926-933

33. Allen IV, McKeown SR (1979) A histological, histochemical and biochemical study of the macroscopically normal white matter in multiple sclerosis. J Neurol Sci 41:81-91

34. Guo AC, Jewells VL, Provenzale JM (2001) Analysis of normal-appearing white matter in multiple sclerosis: comparison of diffusion tensor MR imaging and magnetization transfer imaging. AJNR Am J Neuroradiol 22:1893-1900

35. Guo AC, MacFall JR, Provenzale JM (2002) Multiple sclerosis: diffusion tensor MR imaging for evaluation of normal-appearing white matter. Radiology 222:729-736

36. Thompson AJ, Polman CH, Miller DH et al (1997) Primary progressive multiple sclerosis. Brain 120:1085-1096

37. Cercignani M, Inglese M, Pagani E et al (2001) Mean diffusivity and fractional anisotropy histograms in patients with multiple sclerosis. AJNR Am J Neuroradiol 22:952-958

38. Iannucci G, Rovaris M, Giacomotti L et al (2001) Correlations between measures of

multiple sclerosis pathology derived from T2, T1, magnetization transfer and diffusion tensor MR imaging. AJNR Am J Neuroradiol 22:1462-1467

39. Filippi M, Rocca MA, Martino G et al (1998) Magnetization transfer changes in the normal-appearing white matter precede the appearance of enhancing lesions in patients with multiple sclerosis. Ann Neurol 43:809-814
40. Goodkin DE, Rooney WD, Sloan R et al (1998) A serial study of new MS lesions and the white matter from which they arise. Neurology 51:1689-1697
41. Hajnal JV, Doran M, Hall AS et al (1991) MR imaging of anisotropically restricted diffusion of water in system: technical, anatomic, and pathologic considerations. J Comput Assist Tomogr 15:1-18
42. Peyser JM, Edwards KR, Poser CM, Filskov SB (1980) Cognitive function in patients with multiple sclerosis. Arch Neurol 37:577-579
43. Rovaris M, Iannucci G, Falautano M et al (2002) Cognitive dysfunction in patients with mildly disabling relapsing-remitting multiple sclerosis: an exploratory study with diffusion tensor MR imaging. J Neurol Sci 195:103-109
44. Bozzali M, Cercignani M, Sormani MP et al (2002) Quantification of brain gray matter damage in different MS phenotypes by use of diffusion tensor MR imaging. AJNR Am J Neuroradiol 23:985-988
45. Rovaris M, Bozzali M, Iannucci G et al (2002) Assessment of normal-appearing white and gray matter in patients with primary progressive multiple sclerosis: a diffusion-tensor magnetic resonance imaging study. Arch Neurol 59:1406-1412
46. Filippi M, Bozzali M, Comi G (2001) Magnetization transfer and diffusion tensor MR imaging of basal ganglia from patients with multiple sclerosis. J Neurol Sci 183:69-72
47. Roelcke U, Kappos L, Lechner-Scott J et al (1997) Reduced glucose metabolism in the frontal cortex and basal ganglia of multiple sclerosis patients with fatigue: a ^{18}F-fluorodeoxyglucose positron emission tomography study. Neurology 48:1566-1571
48. Filippi M, Rocca MA, Colombo B et al (2002) Functional magnetic resonance imaging correlates of fatigue in multiple sclerosis. Neuroimage 15:559-567
49. Brück W, Bitsch A, Kolenda H et al (1997) Inflammatory central nervous system demyelination: correlation of magnetic resonance imaging findings with lesion pathology. Ann Neurol 42:783-793
50. van Waesberghe JHTM, Kamphorst W, De Groot CJA (1999) Axonal loss in MS lesions: MR insights into substrates of disability. Ann Neurol 46:747-754
51. Filippi M, Rocca MA, Rizzo G et al (1998) Magnetization transfer ratios in multiple sclerosis lesions enhancing after different doses of gadolinium. Neurology 50:1289-1293
52. Filippi M, Rocca MA, Comi G (1998) Magnetization transfer ratios of multiple sclerosis lesions with variable durations of enhancement. J Neurol Sci 159:162-165
53. Dousset V, Gayou A, Brochet B, Caille JM (1998) Early structural changes in acute MS lesions assessed by serial magnetization transfer studies. Neurology 51:1150-1155
54. Filippi M, Rocca MA, Sormani MP et al (1999) Short-term evolution of individual enhancing MS lesions studied with magnetization transfer imaging. Magn Reson Imaging 17:979-984
55. van Buchem MA, McGowan JC, Kolson DL et al (1996) Quantitative volumetric magnetization transfer analysis in multiple sclerosis: estimation of macroscopic and microscopic disease burden. Magn Reson Med 36:632-636
56. Filippi M, Iannucci G, Tortorella C et al (1999) Comparison of MS clinical phenotypes using conventional and magnetization transfer MRI. Neurology 52:588-594
57. Filippi M, Inglese M, Rovaris M et al (2000) Magnetization transfer imaging to monitor the evolution of MS: a one-year follow up study. Neurology 55:940-946
58. Tortorella C, Viti B, Bozzali M et al (2000) A magnetization transfer histogram study of normal appearing brain tissue in multiple sclerosis. Neurology 54; 186-193

59. Nusbaum AO, Tang CY, Wei TC et al (2000) Whole-brain diffusion MR histograms differ between MS subtypes. Neurology 54:1421-1426

60. Inglese M, Rovaris M, Bianchi S et al (2001) Magnetic resonance imaging, magnetisation transfer imaging and diffusion weighted imaging correlates of optic nerve, brain and cervical cord damage in Leber's hereditary optic neuropathy. J Neurol Neurosurg Psychiatry 70:444-449

61. Inglese M, Salvi F, Iannucci G et al (2002) Magnetization transfer and diffusion tensor MR imaging of acute disseminated encephalomyelitis. AJNR Am J Neuroradiol 23:267-272

62. Castriota Scanderbeg A, Tomaiuolo F, Sabatini U et al (2000) Demyelinating plaques in relapsing-remitting and secondary-progressive multiple sclerosis: assessment with diffusion MR imaging. AJNR Am J Neuroradiol 21:862-868

63. Mainero C, De Stefano N, Iannucci G et al (2001) Correlates of MS disability assessed in-vivo using aggregates of MR quantities. Neurology 56:1331-1334

64. Rocca MA, Falini A, Colombo B et al (2002) Adaptive functional changes in the cerebral cortex of patients with nondisabling multiple sclerosis correlate with the extent of brain structural damage. Ann Neurol 51:330-339

65. Filippi M, Rocca MA, Falini A et al (2002) Correlations between structural CNS damage and functional MRI changes in primary progressive MS. Neuroimage 15:537-546

66. Rocca MA, Matthews PM, Caputo D et al (2002) Evidence for widespread movement-associated functional MRI changes in patients with PPMS. Neurology 58:866-872

67. Mori S, Crain BJ, Chacko VP, van Zijl PC (1999) Three-dimensional tracking of axonal projections in the brain by magnetic resonance imaging. Ann Neurol 45:265-269

68. Mori S, Kaufmann WE, Davatzikos C et al (2002) Imaging cortical association tracts in the human brain using diffusion-tensor-based axonal tracking. Magn Reson Med 47:215-223

69. Conturo TE, Lori NF, Cull TS et al (1999) Tracking neuronal fiber pathways in the living human brain. Proc Natl Acad Sci U S A 96:10422-10427

70. Tench CR, Morgan PS, Wilson M, Blumhardt LD (2002) White matter mapping using diffusion tensor MRI. Magn Reson Med 47:967-972

71. Iwasawa T, Matoba H, Ogi A et al (1997) Diffusion-weighted imaging of the human optic nerve: a new approach to evaluate optic neuritis in multiple sclerosis. Magn Reson Med 38:484-491

72. Wheeler-Kingshott CA, Parker GJM, Symms MR et al (2002) ADC mapping of the human optic nerve: increased resolution, coverage, and reliability with CSF-suppressed ZOOM-EPI. Magn Reson Med 47:24-31

73. Clark CA, Werring DJ, Miller DH (2000) Diffusion imaging of the spinal cord in vivo: estimation of the principal diffusivities and application to multiple sclerosis. Magn Reson Med 43:133-138

74. Ries M, Jones RA, Dousset V, Moonen CTW (2000) Diffusion tensor MRI of the spinal cord. Magn Reson Med 44:884-892

75. Bammer R, Fazekas F, Augustin M et al (2000) Diffusion-weighted MR imaging of the spinal cord. AJNR Am J Neuroradiol 21:587-591

76. Robertson RL, Maier SE, Mulkern RV et al (2000) MR line-scan diffusion imaging of the spinal cord in children. AJNR Am J Neuroradiol 21:1344-1348

77. Wheeler-Kingshott CA, Hickman SJ, Parker GJ et al (2002) Investigating cervical spinal cord structure using axial diffusion tensor imaging. Neuroimage 16:93-102

78. Bammer R, Augustin M, Prokesch RW et al (2002) Diffusion-weighted imaging of the spinal cord: interleaved echo-planar imaging is superior to fast spin-echo. J Magn Reson Imaging 15:364-373

Chapter 4

Global Brain Proton MR Spectroscopy in MS

O. Gonen, R.I. Grossman

Introduction

Multiple sclerosis (MS) is the most common demyelinating disease of the central nervous system, affecting nearly 350 000 Americans, 100 000 Britons, and over 2 million people worldwide. It is the leading cause of nontraumatic neurological disability in young and middle-aged adults [1]. Roughly 85% of MS patients, two-thirds of whom are women, experience acute symptoms over short (weeks) periods, followed by variable, unpredictable lengths (months to years) of partial or complete remission, entering the relapsing-remitting (RR) stage. These cycles continue, leading to accumulating clinical disability from incomplete remissions. After 10 years, 50% will enter the secondary progressive phase of the disease [2]. This progression entails chronic clinical deterioration, increasing motor, sensory, and cognitive deficits, but not a significant reduction of life expectancy [2].

Although T1- and T2-weighted MRI have greatly improved our ability to detect macroscopic MS pathology, becoming the foremost tool for paraclinical diagnosis and treatment efficacy monitoring [3], they lack pathological specificity and sensitivity to microscopic occult pathology [4]. Postmortem studies have shown MS pathogenesis to include inflammation and/or demyelination, axonal loss, and gliosis, not only in lesions, which comprise less than 5% of the brain volume [5], but also in normal-appearing tissue [6].

This diffuse pathogenesis in the normal-appearing white matter (NAWM) leads to global neuronal and axonal damage [7, 8], which persists even during periods of clinical remission, as reflected by the formation of new lesions and enlargement of old ones [9]. Although this activity may play a central role in the evolution of MS from its earlier RR to its secondary progressive phase [10], it is invisible to conventional imaging. To investigate such occult processes, quantitative techniques, such as magnetization transfer imaging (MTI), proton MR spectroscopy (^{1}H-MRS), and diffusion tensor imaging (DTI), have been used [4]. All have shown that changes in the NAWM may (1) precede lesion formation [11-13], (2) occur in all MS phenotypes [14-17], and (3) correlate with physical disability and cognitive impairment [16-20].

It has recently been suggested that axonal damage followed by neuronal cell death by wallerian degeneration is the probable cause of permanent neurological deficits in MS [21, 22]. This can be assessed directly by ^{1}H-MRS quantification of the amino-acid derivative N-acetylaspartate (NAA) [23, 24], found almost exclusively in neurons and axons [25-27]. Its loss in lesions has been detected by ¹H-MRS [23, 28, 29] and established directly by histopathological methods [30-32]. Unfortunately, the single-voxel or single-slice 2D ¹H-MRS methods used restricted the volumes of interest (VOI), rendering most of the NAWM status invisible not only to the MRI but to ¹H-MRS as well [7, 33]. Therefore, NAA assessment of the entire parenchyma is crucial to evaluate the full extent of the disease. Indeed, a new ¹H-MRS method to quantify the whole-brain NAA (WBNAA) concentration has recently shown that the latter can be more than 20% lower in RRMS patients than in their healthy contemporaries, and declines ten times faster with age [7, 34].

The need for effective prognostic markers for MS coupled with the direct link established between the disease, axonal loss, and NAA deficits motivated the studies outlined in this chapter into the amount(s) and rate(s) of metabolite abnormality evolution in absolute terms and as functions of disease duration. The rationale was that, given limited resources, patients and clinical trial candidates should be preselected for treatment based on the best available estimates of their current disease severity and its predicted future course [35-37].

WBNAA Evidence for Different Clinical Cohorts

The high interpatient variability of clinical symptoms and poor prediction of disease course make markers of disease activity that could identify a high risk of early rapid deterioration and the optimal treatment regimen highly desirable. This took on a new urgency during the 1990s, when, after nearly 150 years in which MS has been diagnosed, several long-term therapies have received FDA approval in the US, e.g., interferon beta-1a (Avonex), interferon beta-1b (Betaseron), and copolymer-1 (Copaxone) [38-40]. However, at an approximate annual cost of $ 15 000 per patient [41], spending in the US alone exceeds $2.5 billion per year [42]. Consequently, outside the US, the cost/benefit of the drugs is controversial and treatment is not universally offered. In the UK, for example, interferon is administered to only 3% of patients [43].

Considering the early age of onset, disease duration, the cost of treatment, its side effects, and inconvenience, both patient and neurologist face three central questions [35]: (1) What is the disease's probable long-term course? (2) Is its activity severe enough to need therapeutic intervention? (3) What is the efficacy of therapy? Unfortunately, there are currently no reliable prognostic indices as clinical and cognitive measures do not predict future course [44-46]. Laboratory markers of disease progression, such as oligoclonal bands, have been only moderately useful and are invasive [47]. MRI methods, although diagnostic for individuals experiencing a clinical event but not yet confirmed as having clinically definite (CD) MS [48, 49], provide little prognostic information due to the variable course and pathological heterogeneity of the disease [9, 50].

Materials and Methods

Patients

Forty-nine patients with RRMS were studied. None was undergoing a relapse at the time of examination. Their CD disease duration (ΔY), prior to WBNAA acquisition, was defined as

$$\Delta Y = (\text{date of WBNAA scan}) - (\text{date of CD diagnosis}). \qquad (1)$$

Gender, average disease duration, and Expanded Disability Status Scale (EDSS) details of this cohort are summarized in Table 1. All participating subjects gave their Institutional Review Board-approved written consent.

WBNAA Quantification

The amount of NAA in the whole brain, Q_{NAA}, was obtained in a 4-T Signa wholebody imager with its standard head coil (GE Medical Systems, Milwaukee, Wis). Our high (third)-order auto-shim procedure yielded consistent 30 ± 5 Hz fullwidth-at-half-maximum whole-head water linewidth. A nonlocalizing, nonecho ^{1}H-MRS followed to obtain the whole-head NAA signal, as described previously [34]. The entire procedure required approximately 25 min. Absolute quantification was done with a phantom replacement reference 3-l sphere of 15 mmol NAA in water. Subject and reference NAA peak areas, S_S and S_P, were integrated and Q_{NAA} calculated as [34]

$$Q_{NAA} = (1.5 \times 10^{-2}) \times S_S/S_P \, (P_S^{180°}/P_P^{180°})^{1/2} \text{ moles.} \qquad (2)$$

$P_P^{180°}$ and $P_S^{180°}$ are the transmitter power into 50 Ω for a nonselective, 1-ms 180° inversion pulse on the phantom and subject respectively, and reflect the momentary system's sensitivity.

To address the natural variations in brain sizes, Q_{NAA} was divided by the subject's brain volume, V_B, obtained from high-resolution MRI at 1.5 T (256^2 matrix, 220 mm^2 FOV, 3-mm-thick slices, proton density and T_2-weighted fast spin echo, $TE_1/TE_2/TR = 16/80/2500$ ms). The images were processed with the 3DVIEWNIX package, which, based on several manually preselected intensity points in the CSF

Table 1. Summary data of the 49 patients with RRMS grouped according to average rate of decline of WBNAA (see pp 51-52)

	"Stable"	"Moderate"	"Rapid"
Number (M/F)	10 (3/7)	27 (8/19)	12 (5/7)
Age (years): mean (range)	38 (30–50)	40 (24–55)	37 (25–46)
ΔY (years)[a]: mean (range)	6.6 (0.25–22)	7.6 (1–11.5)	0.98 (0.08–6.3)
EDSS[b]: mean (range)	2.0 (1.5–3.5)	2.0 (0.0–6.0)	2.0 (0.0–3.5)

[a] ΔY, Disease duration (see Eq. 1)
[b] EDSS, Expanded Disability Status Scale [79], within 6 months of the WBNAA scan

and gray and white matter, creates a brain mask [51]. V_B is the sum of the pixels within this mask. The method has shown better than 99% reproducibility [52]. Finally the WBNAA concentration, $WBNAA$, was defined as

$$WBNAA = Q_{NAA}/V_B,\qquad(3)$$

suitable for intersubject cross-sectional comparisons.

Statistical Analysis

A previous study of nine female and four male controls, 16-52 years old, estimated their average ± standard-deviation (σ) $WBNAA$ to be 13.2 ± 0.6 mM [7]. Thus, by comparison, the i-th patient's average rate of $WBNAA$ decline per year of disease, $\bar{R}_i$, was estimated to be

$$\bar{R}_i = (13,2 - WBNAA_i)/\Delta Y \text{ mM/year},\qquad(4)$$

where $WBNAA_i$ is the i-th patient's NAA concentration after ΔY_i years of disease as defined by Eq. 1. It is important to point out that Eq. 4 implicitly assumes that the $WBNAA$ loss relative to "normal" (13.2 ± 0.6 mM) started either at or, at most, very shortly before diagnosis.

The 49 patients were divided into subgroups based on their $\bar{R}_i$, as described below. Least-squares regression was used to assess the relationship of $WBNAA$ with ΔY and age in each group. Since the groups were constructed based on estimated $\bar{R}_i$, they could not be meaningfully cross-compared with regard to their average rate of $WBNAA$ decline. Furthermore, since only 11 patients were on immunomodulatory treatment of various types and length, either in absolute terms or as a percentage of disease duration, this factor was excluded from the analyses.

Results

WBNAA correlation with disease duration

Annual WBNAA Decline Rates

The $\bar{R}_i$s of Eq. 4 for the 49 patients are plotted in Fig. 1. Since a previous study of 13 controls has shown their $WBNAA$ to be statistically constant with age [7], the ten patients whose $\bar{R}_i \leq 0$ mM/year were defined as "stable" in Fig. 1b. Since the reproducibility of $WBNAA$ was shown to have $\sigma = 0.6$ mM [34], the 12 individuals exhibiting $\bar{R}_i \geq 3\sigma$/year (1.7 mM/year) were deemed to be significantly different from "stable" and defined as suffering a "rapid" decline. The bulk (27) of the cohort, for whom $0 \leq \bar{R}_i \leq 1.7$ mM/year, were defined as undergoing "moderate" decline, as shown in Fig. 1b.

WBNAA Versus Disease Duration

The patients' WBNAA level versus ΔY from Eq. 1, are plotted in Fig. 2. The symbolic labels for each patient were determined by their group assignment as

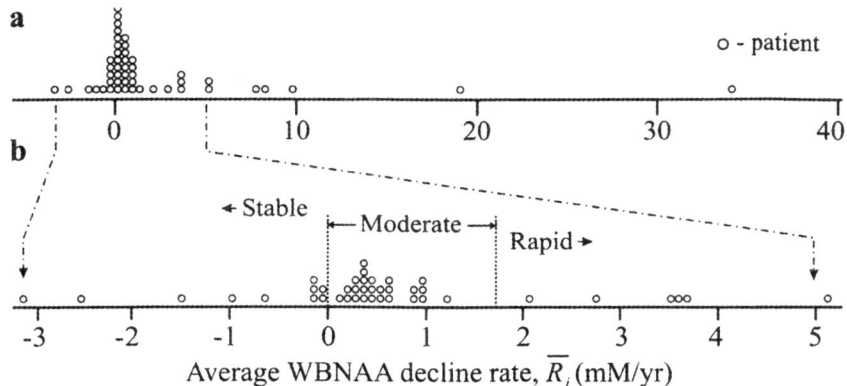

Fig. 1. a Dot-plot of the individual patients' (μ) distribution as a function of their average rate of WBNAA decline per year of disease duration ($\bar{R}_i$), as defined by Eqs. 1 and 4. **b** Expanded – 3 to + 5 mM/year region of **a**. The *vertical dotted* lines at $\bar{R}_i = 0$ and 1.7 mM/year partition the group according to criteria defined in the text

described above and shown in Fig. 1b. It is striking that although Fig. 1 exhibits a nearly continuous distribution, Fig. 2 readily exhibits three distinct subgroups, without any further assumptions or postprocessing.

Least-squares regression was used to characterize the cross-sectional associa-

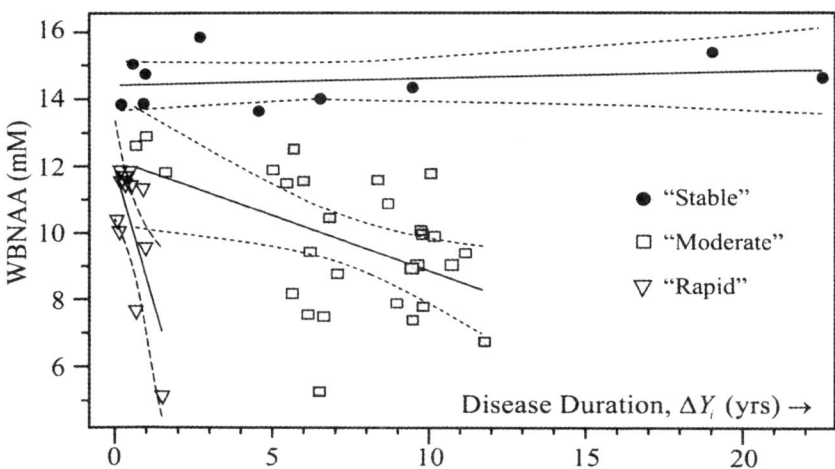

Fig. 2. Individuals' WBNAA levels as a function of their disease duration: ΔY of Eq. 1. The groupings: "Stable" (●) "Moderate" (□) and "Rapid" (▽) were determined as described in the text. ■ indicates patients receiving medication at the time of the measurement (all "Moderate"). *Solid lines* are the regression for each subgroup (Eqs. 5-7) and the *dashed lines* are their ±95% confidence intervals

tion between WBNAA and ΔY in the subgroups. It showed that for the "stable" group the linear relationship was

$$WBNAA_S = 14.37 + 0.02 \times \Delta Y \; [mM], \tag{5}$$

where $WBNAA_S$ is the predicted concentration for a patient whose disease duration, ΔY years, is defined by Eq. 1. Similarly, the linear prediction equation for the "moderate" group was

$$WBNAA_M = 12.18 - 0.34 \times \Delta Y \; [mM], \tag{6}$$

and for the "rapid" group,

$$WBNAA_R = 12.14 - 3.39 \times \Delta Y \; [mM]. \tag{7}$$

Specifically, "stable" patients exhibited an insignificant increase of 0.02 mM/year ($p = 0.54$) whereas the "moderate" and "rapid" subgroups suffered significant average WBNAA loss of 0.34 and 3.39 mM/year ($p = 0.001$ and 0.001), respectively.

To assess whether a linear model best predicts the WBNAA behavior within each rate group, least-squares polynomial regression was also performed. The model function included terms up to cubic in disease duration. In every subgroup, however, neither the cubic nor quadratic terms were found to be statistically significant ($p > 0.19$).

Expressing these annual changes as a percentage of the intercept in Eqs. 5-7 yields 0%, – 2.8%, and – 27.9% for the subgroups, in order. The regression lines of Eqs. 5-7, together with their respective $\pm$ 95% confidence intervals (CI), are also plotted in Fig. 2. The median disease durations of the "stable" and "moderate" subgroups were not significantly different ($p = 0.11$) but both were longer ($p < 0.01$) than for the "rapid" subgroup.

WBNAA Correlation with Patient Age

No significant correlation between age and WBNAA was found for any subgroup.

WBNAA Correlation with EDSS Scores

Spearman rank correlation coefficients were produced to test the within-group relationship between WBNAA and EDSS scores. Mann-Whitney analyses were used to test for differences between the groups' EDSS scores. These scores were not significantly different between any of the groups (cf. Table 1). The cohort's WBNAA did not correlate with EDSS ($p > 0.05$). Between-group correlation was inappropriate as the groups are the result of a statistical construct.

Discussion

Reduced NAA in the lesions and NAWM of MS patients has been shown by ^{1}H-MRS for the past decade [23, 29, 53, 54]. However, unequivocal connection between MS, axonal loss, and NAA deficits has only recently been established by

Bjartmar et al. from immunopathology and immunocytochemistry on post-mortem spinal cord samples from lesions and NAWM of MS patients and from white matter in their matched deceased controls [31]. Patients' lower axonal density and proportionally lower NAA/unit-volume were both shown to correlate with neurological impairment [31]. Previously, Trapp et al. used similar methods to demonstrate that axonal loss in acute and chronic cerebral MS lesions correlated with NAA reduction [30]. Thus, WBNAA deficit is a direct noninvasively measured indicator of total axonal loss, which in turn reflects the pathological load of the disease.

This study provides evidence for the existence of three differential strata of axonal loss in 49 clinically similar RRMS patients (cf. average EDSS scores in Table 1), based on cross-sectional rate of *WBNAA* decline as a function of disease duration (cf. Fig. 2). This indicates that, despite clinical similarity, these patients sustained disparate levels of axonal loss accumulated at different rates. Specifically, a "stable" group, comprising 20% of the cohort, exhibited constant WBNAA levels, similar to those of matched controls [7]. A second subgroup comprising the majority (55%) of the patients sustained a "moderate" 0.34 mM/year or 2.7% loss. Compared with them, the remaining 25% suffered a ten-fold more "rapid" decline and their median disease duration was significantly shorter than that of either of the other two groups, as seen from Table 1 and Fig. 2.

No subgroup exhibited a correlation between *WBNAA* decline and patients' age. Together with absolute WBNAA levels at or above "normal" (13.2 ± 0.6 mM) (cf. Fig. 2), this reflects maintenance of neuronal integrity in the "stable" group. The "rapid" group's *WBNAA* did not correlate with age either, but their low WBNAA levels suggest that they represent a different, aggressive variant of MS that can onset at any age, not a form of "moderate" disease that suddenly accelerated. Furthermore, this study indicates that the decline observed in two of the three groups (cf. Fig. 2), and in the majority of patients, is on average a continual one-way process. Therefore, even if local, or even global, repair and recovery is possible, as suggested recently [24, 55, 56], it may be only partial and temporary. The long-term trend of MS is a global average decline, as is to be expected from a chronic degenerative disease.

Since WBNAA offers an evaluation of the entire brain, deviations from "normal" reflect the current total axonal deficit, and its rate of decline is an index of disease aggression. In this study, patients had their WBNAA measured only once; hence, the rates reported are cross-sectional, not derived from serial follow-ups. Nevertheless, this does not detract from these results' general utility, especially since current medical practice requires two separate clinical episodes to confirm MS.

This study suggests that *WBNAA* should be evaluated upon presentation of the first neurological symptom for three reasons:

1. A deficit compared with the 13.2 ± 0.6 mM average "normal" could indicate developing pathology [54]. This is demonstrated in Fig. 2, where all "moderate" and "rapid" patients exhibit *below*-normal *WBNAA*.
2. If (or when) these individuals present with another clinical episode, a second WBNAA evaluation at that time would establish their *individual* rate of axon-

al loss, facilitating subgroup assignment upon disease confirmation. Alternatively, as it is common for patients to go several years between first and second relapses, it may be appropriate to schedule a second WBNAA scan 1 year after the initial event – a common interval for patient consultations. Considering the prognostic and treatment-staging consequences of belonging to the "rapid" subgroup [18], described below, it is imperative that this assignment be as accurate as possible.

3. Children of two parents with MS or with female siblings who have contracted the disease at an early age (21 years or earlier) are at a very high (30%) risk of developing the disease themselves [57-60]. Such substantial identifiable risk, combined with relatively small numbers of prospective candidates in the general population, may merit screening for developing subclinical symptoms. This is especially germane considering the availability of approved medications and their known ability to forestall conversion of monosymptomatic episodes to CD MS [36, 37].

The disparity between the patients' clinical similarity and their WBNAA levels and dynamics reflects the brain's ability to compensate for accumulating injury and conceal its extent. This plasticity underlies the difficulty of using clinical criteria such as EDSS to predict disease course. While a useful clinical measure of neurological impairment, EDSS consistently fails to reflect the full burden of the disease, due to its weighting toward cerebellar and spinal cord deficits [44, 50]. In contrast, *WBNAA* yields the cerebral pathological load directly, and its inferred rate of change in the "moderate" and "rapid" groups well exceeds the ~1%/year. reported for global atrophy [61, 62]. Therefore, we hypothesize that the subgroup dynamics presented here predict future maintenance of clinical function and, therefore, could establish (1) long-term prognosis, (2) treatment priority, and (3) more effective candidate selection criterion for clinical trials.

Prognosis

A major concern for newly diagnosed patients is the future course of their disease. As yet, no clinical or paraclinical measure provides a definitive forecast. Scott et al. isolated six indices for age, symptoms, MRI status, intervals between first and second attacks, frequency of episodes in the first 2 years, and completeness of recovery [63]. Patients classed as "high risk" for four or more indices were found to have significantly greater disease progression and lower EDSS scores. However, they comprised only 24% of the cohort, underscoring the difficulty of assigning prognosis. In contrast, *WBNAA* dynamics may provide a noninvasive prognostic measure for *all* patients. Specifically, "stable" patients may anticipate decades of little accumulation of cerebral pathology (cf. Fig. 2), and hence no need for therapeutic intervention. The majority of patients, those exhibiting "moderate" decline, may expect to follow the established model of MS progression with its 10- and 20-year disability landmarks [2]. Indeed, due perhaps to their clinically recognized course and duration, the 11 patients on a medication while in this study were all in that group. Finally, those in the "rapid" subgroup should perhaps be advised, despite a short disease duration, of the increased likelihood of decline in their quality of life [2, 18, 54], and encouraged to engage in aggressive treatment to forestall it [36, 37].

Staging Treatment

Criteria for treatment of MS vary from country to country. Enrollment into therapeutic regimens is usually determined by clinical status, age, general health, acceptance of injection regimen, and, increasingly, funding. This study suggests that clinically similar RRMS patients accumulate axonal pathology at significantly different rates. Therefore, their *WBNAA* dynamics may provide the sought-after noninvasive indication for staging treatment. Specifically, it may be beneficial to start medication in the most rapidly declining population (righthand side of Fig. 1) and proceed to include more patients as far leftwards towards "stable" on that axis as the available resources will allow [36].

Stratification for Clinical Trials

It is ethically unacceptable to conduct a prospective treatment of unknown efficacy when proven ones are available. Therefore, since new drug trials must use the least number of patients for the shortest period of time, induction based on pathological rather than clinical disease status could raise their efficiency. Different levels of pathology and dynamics, shown here to exist in the general RRMS population, could confound phase II and III clinical trials with type I and II statistical errors [64]. Type I errors may be encountered when "stable" patients favorably bias finding to show an ineffective drug as efficacious. The more detrimental type II errors could be incurred when "rapid" patients erroneously cause rejection of an effective drug due to inadequate response. Considering the cost of pharmaceutical development, these could be expensive mistakes [64]. Consequently, randomized recruitment based entirely on clinical metrics such as EDSS will necessitate larger sample sizes and longer durations to achieve a given statistical power [37, 65], than homogeneous "moderate" or "rapid" cohorts selected based on *WBNAA* dynamics.

WBNAA may, in addition, allow monitoring of the neuroprotective ability of a putative treatment, since it is possible to measure global NAA deficit at presentation and the rate of its loss serially over time. This would indicate the individual patient's neuronal integrity at the start, during, and at the end points of drug studies. However, an intrinsic limitation of the WBNAA approach is that it is insensitive to spinal cord pathology. Thus, patients with predominantly spinal disease may be given an incorrect positive prognosis. The clinical effect of spinal lesions can be significant, either through specific damage to sensitive areas or by causing wallerian degeneration "upstream" into the brain [22].

Prospects of Staging Treatment Based on WBNAA

Upon diagnosis, both patient and clinician are faced with the questions of prognosis and disease management [35], especially considering the availability of approved treatment [39, 40, 66], which provides RR and SP patients effective therapeutic regimes known to reduce disease progression [38]. Unfortunately, since these therapies are controversial because of their limited efficacy and annual cost per individual, (US$ 12-15 000 [41]), they are offered to less than 25% of MS patients within the various European national health care systems [67]. Considering these constraints, therapy decisions should be based on a patient's prognosis. Unfortunately, this cannot be forecast with enough reliability due to the variable course of the disease. Clinical markers, such as EDSS and cognitive function, are not predictive of the future disease course [45, 46]; neither are para-clinical markers of disease load such as MRI [9, 50] or oligoclonal bands, found in the cerebrospinal fluid, which are only slightly more reliable but are invasive [47].

Trapp et al. have shown that axonal transection is a feature of both acute and chronic MS lesions [30], while Bjartmar et al. demonstrated that axonal loss correlates to NAA decline and such permanent deficits relate to neurological disability [31]. Therefore, WBNAA, which reflects the global disease volume, could potentially be a better metric of the overall pathological load in an individual. Furthermore, as axonal loss leads to permanent functional deficit, its assessment at onset may indicate the extent/aggressiveness of early disease activity.

To test this hypothesis we investigated the degree of axonal loss in a group of patients just (within the past year) diagnosed with RRMS. The aim was to ascertain whether, in such a clinically homogeneous, low-EDSS group, different levels of WBNAA loss exist at the earliest stage in their initial (RR) phase of the disease. Such information could be used to identify those who have accumulated the greatest neurological injury and therefore need prioritized management.

Materials and methods

Patients

Fifteen patients with CD RRMS diagnosed within the last year were studied. Their caracteristics are summarized in Table 2. None was on any immunomodulatory medication regimen or was undergoing a relapse at the time of WBNAA quantification. Their EDSS was measured within 6 months of scanning. The experiment was approved by the Institutional Review Board and all participating subjects gave their written informed consent. The WBNAA measurement carried out is identical to the one outlined on pp. 49-50, above.

Results

WBNAA Concentrations

The WBNAA concentration of each of the 15 patients is plotted in Fig. 3. A previous study of 13 healthy controls (see p. 50, above) has shown their average concentration to be 13.2 mM, statistically stable with age, indicated by the arrow in Fig. 3 [7]. Its reproducibility analysis has shown that there is 99% confidence that a subject is different from this average if his or her WBNAA concentration is more

Table 2. Descriptive statistics of the 15 patients with RRMS studied

Variable	Value
Number (M/F)	15 (5/10)
Age (years): mean (range)	36.8 (25.0-46.4)
WBNAA (mM): mean (range)	11.9 (7.6-15.0)
EDSS: mean (range)	2 (1.5-3.5)

than 3 standard deviations, σ, =1.7 mM [34]. Consequently, the region of "normal" $\pm 3\sigma$ is highlighted on Fig. 3 and patients whose WBNAA concentration fell within that range were deemed to be indistinguishable from healthy individuals, i.e., deemed to have suffered no NAA loss at the current stage of their disease. In contrast, the six individuals (40% of the present study population) who fell outside that range have all suffered a statistically significant NAA loss of variable severity and are clearly abnormal.

Correlation of WBNAA Concentration with Patient Age

No significant correlation was found between age and WBNAA.

Correlation of WBNAA Concentration with EDSS Scores

WBNAA concentration did not correlate with EDSS ($p > 0.05$).

Discussion

RR disease is the prevailing form of MS, with a 2:1 female:male ratio and a 27-year-old mean age of onset in the US [1]. Its sufferers initially have mild levels of disability that do not preclude continued social and professional function including pregnancy. For clinicians, these are the patients with whom they have the greatest involvement, as the patients are at the start of their disease process and

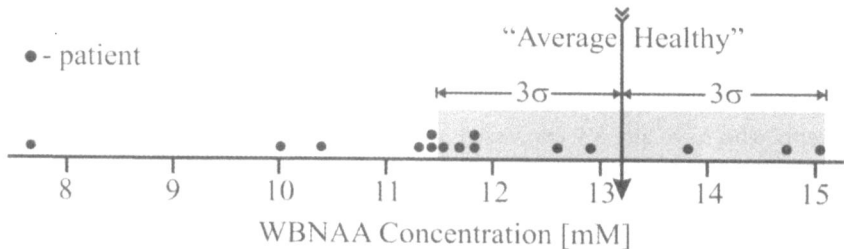

Fig. 3. Dot-plot of the 15 MS patients (●) distribution as a function of their WBNAA concentration within 1 year of clinical confirmation of the diagnosis. The *vertical arrow* indicates the average concentration, 13.2 mM, found in healthy individuals in the 18-53 years of age range. The *shaded region* indicates the $\pm 3\sigma$ (± 1.7 mM) of the "normal" span

are anxious to take whatever steps are available or possible to slow their disease and relieve its symptoms [35].

In the last decade immunomodulating drugs such as interferon-β have became available for effective clinical management. Patient selection for such treatments currently depends upon meeting criteria of clinical disability, age, frequency of relapse, and ability to sustain the subcutaneous administration procedures and its side effects. In addition, financial constraints are imposed on the administration of such expensive, potentially very long-term treatment, especially since not all patients benefit equally from it. Therefore, selection for treatment would benefit from markers that will identify, (1) who has already accumulated significant enough pathology to require prioritized intervention and (2) who might respond favorably, not only with reduced frequency of relapses, but, perhaps more importantly, with a slowing or a complete halt of their WBNAA decline [35].

This study demonstrates that a cohort of clinically homogeneous RRMS patients (EDSS 1.5-3.5, see Table 2) already exhibits a broad distribution of WBNAA levels in the earliest stages of the disease, as shown in Fig. 3. This may indicate that quantifiable neuronal damage, of variable severity, already exists as early as (and probably before) the confirmed diagnosis in some but not all patients. Differentiating such patients according to the deviation of their WBNAA level from "average healthy," as depicted in Fig. 3, may provide the neurologist with an additional objective, instrumental, and, as importantly, noninvasive criterion for patient stratification for treatment based on pathological rather than purely clinical grounds: specifically, to start with the leftmost patient on the WBNAA axis of Fig. 3 and proceed towards the right selecting patients till all available treatment resources are exhausted.

The efficacy of current therapies is a source of constant debate and review, since, although proven to be beneficial, their effect has not been consistent across patient groups. When a reduction in disease progression following treatment is achieved, it is sometimes not as great as one would desire. Such apparent lack of a clinical effect may reflect either an ineffective drug or inability of a patient to respond due to having already sustained significant neuronal cell losses. Since WBNAA quantification evaluates the entire brain, it is an assessment of the global volume of the disease, which may provide a predictor of what level of response can best be expected.

Assigning prognosis on the basis of the data presented here would be premature. However, it seems rational to hypothesize that these newly diagnosed patients who have already expressed significant NAA loss may undergo clinical deterioration sooner than those who exhibit relative neuronal stability compared with the average of the controls (see Fig. 3). In addition, acquisition of WBNAA concentration at intervals of standard clinical follow-up would enable clinicians to monitor the progress of the disease and, for the patients on drug therapies, could indicate the effectiveness of the latter. This capability may become even more prominent with the development of neuroprotecting medications for MS in addition to or instead of the current anti-inflammatory drugs.

Finally, an intrinsic limitation of the WBNAA approach should also be noted: since it examines only the brain, it is impervious to spinal cord pathology. Thus, patients with predominantly spinal cord disease may be assessed overoptimistically. The clinical effect of spinal lesions can be significant, either through specific damage to eloquent areas, or by causing wallerian degeneration "upstream" into the brain.

Creatine and Choline: the "Other" Metabolites

Since the mid 1980s, MRI has shown MS activity, as reflected by lesion formation, to persist during remission at approximately tenfold the relapse pace [9]. Furthermore, triple-contrast-dose MRI reveals on average 70% more enhancing lesions, suggesting that extensive low-grade inflammation goes undetected [4]. Indeed, ^{1}H-MRS, MTI, DTI, and segmentation have all shown continual activity in the NAWM, which correlated with the degree and progression of disability. [4] Postmortem studies showed this activity to comprise microglial activation, axonal injury, inflammation, de- and re-myelination, astrocytic proliferation, and atrophy [6, 30, 31, 68].

Since its introduction to MS by Arnold et al. [69], ^{1}H-MRS studies focused on the NAA signal due to its direct connections to axonal dysfunction [7, 30, 70]. However, variable elevation of choline (Cho)/creatine (Cr) and free lipid levels have also been reported, both in acute lesions and in NAWM [16, 71-75], and interpreted as fluctuations in membrane turnover rates due to the inflammation/demyelination processes [32]. Present in both neurons and glial cells, [Cho] and [Cr] were shown to be much higher in astrocytes and oligodendrocytes of cell culture extracts [76]. Unfortunately, the single-voxel or single-slice 2D ^{1}H-MRS methods used restricted the volumes of interest (VOIs), rendering most of the NAWM status invisible not only to the MRI but to ^{1}H-MRS as well [7, 33].

In this section we aim to assess the metabolic characteristics in a more comprehensive volume of NAWM in RR MS patients. Towards this end we compared the concentrations [NAA], [Cho], and [Cr] between MS patients and their matched controls, in order to test the following hypotheses: (1) that de- and/or re-myelinating processes are diffusely active, even during clinical remission; (2) that this activity is reflected by [Cho] and [Cr] abnormalities; and (3) the end-stage indicators for the pathogenesis are axonal damage, reflected by NAA loss, and atrophy. Since Cho and Cr are present in all tissue types, the whole-brain approach proposed for NAA, which is intrinsically localized to neuronal cells [7, 34], is inappropriate. To address that issue as well as the limited VOIs examined in previous studies, we resorted to 3D ^{1}H-MRS in order to cover a substantial 480-cm^3 region of mostly white matter, centered about the corpus callosum, as shown in Fig. 4 [77].

Materials and Methods

Subjects

Eleven patients (8 women, 3 men), mean age 39 (range 26-48) years and 9 healthy subjects (7 women, 2 men), mean age 32 (range 21-48) years, were recruited for this study. The former had CD RRMS [78] for a median duration of 6.9 (range 3.9-10.9) years and median Expanded Disability Status Scale (EDSS) [79] score of 2.5 (range 0.0-6.0). No patient had a relapse during the study or the preceding 3 months and 8 of the 11 were on immunomodulatory drugs. All subjects were briefed on the procedure they were about to undertake and gave their Institutional Review Board approved written informed consent.

MRI, 3D ¹H-MRS, and Metabolite Quantification

All experiments were done in a 1.5-T Magnetom 63SP (Siemens AG, Erlangen, Germany). Axial, sagittal and coronal T1-weighted (T1W) spin-echo (TE/TR = 15/450 ms) MR images were obtained at 240^2 mm field of view and 256^2 matrices. Auto-shimming followed to yield 6.0 ± 1.0 Hz full-width-at-half-maximum water lines from the VOI [80]. Then, a 3D ¹H-MRS sequence with TE/TR =135/1600 ms excited an image-guided 8 cm left-right (LR) × 10 cm anterior-posterior (AP) × 6 cm inferior-superior (IS) = 480 cm³ VOI (cf. Fig. 4) partitioned with 1D-eight-order Hadamard hybrid with 2D $16_{LR} \times 16_{AP}$ chemical shift imaging, into $8_{LR} \times 10_{AP} \times 8_{IS} = 640$ voxels, $1.0_{LR} \times 1.0_{AP} \times 0.75_{IS} = 0.75$ cm³ each [77]. The entire protocol took less than 80 min.

Residual water was removed from the ¹H-MRS data in the time domain; the signals were apodized with a 2 Hz lorentzian, 2D voxel-shifted to align the chemical shift imaging grid with the VOI, Fourier transformed along the LR, AP, and time directions, and Hadamard transformed along the IS orientation [77]. Automatic frequency, zero-th (and first) order phase corrections were made using NAA (and Cho) peaks for reference in voxels where either (or both) were present.

Relative amounts of the i-th (= NAA, Cr, or Cho) metabolite in the j-th voxel of the k-th subject, Q_{ijk}, were estimated from their spectral peak areas, S_{ijk}, using parametric spectral modeling and least-squares optimization [81]. The Q_{ijk}s were scaled into absolute amounts by repeating the 3D experiment on a reference $V_R = 3$ L sphere of 0.033 moles of NAA in water [82],

$$Q_{ijk} \approx \frac{S_{ijk} \times V_V}{S_R \times V_R} \times \sqrt{\frac{P_k^{180°}}{P_R^{180°}}} \times 0.033 \text{ moles,} \tag{8}$$

where $\bar{S}_p$ is the reference's average voxelar NAA peak area and V_V the voxel volume. $P_k^{180°}$ and $P_R^{180°}$ are the powers needed for nonselective, 1-ms inversion pulses on the subject and reference, reflecting their relative "receive" sensitivity. Although possible regional T1 or T2 variations were ignored [83], subsequent analyses are still consistent since similar anatomies are compared.

A VOI centered on the corpus callosum includes ventricular spaces filled with metabolite-free CSF [84]. To account for its volume variation, especially amongst

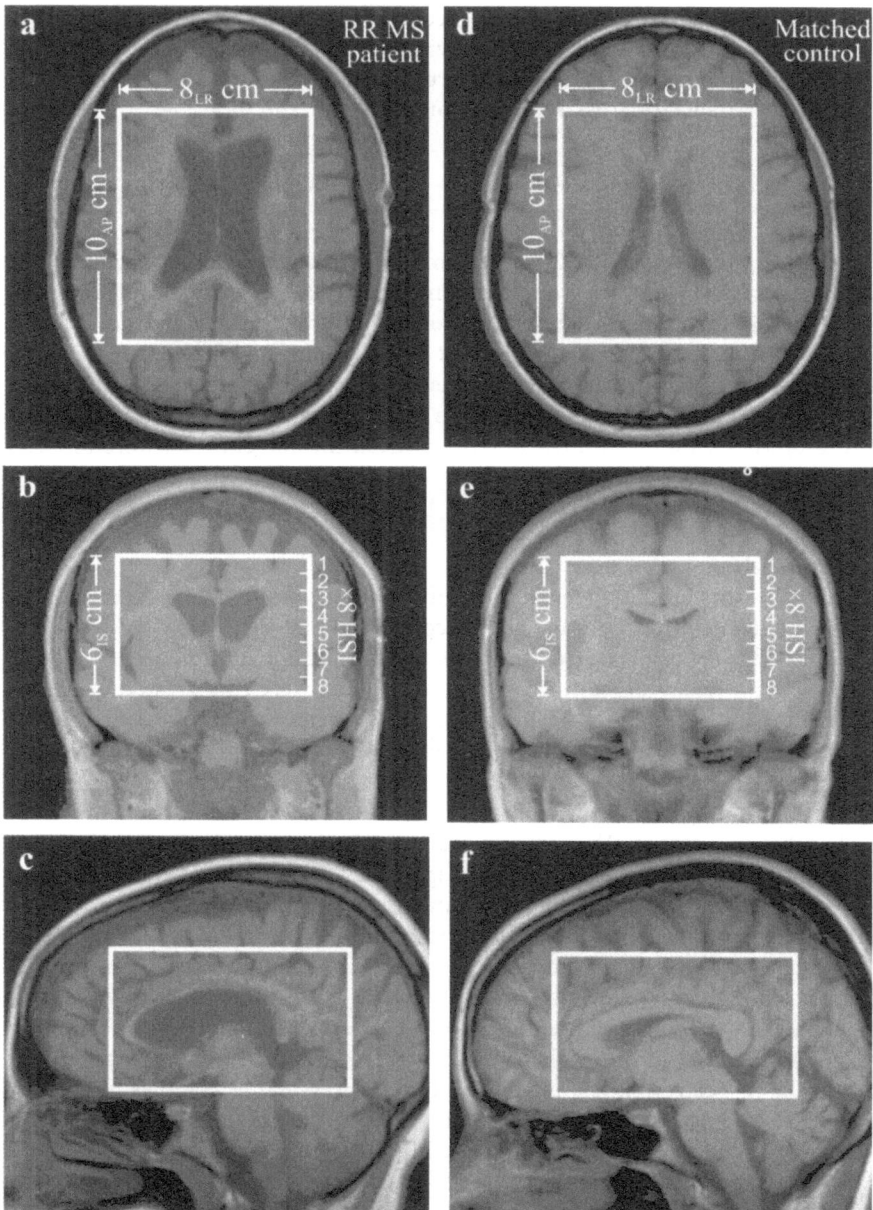

Fig. 4. a-c Axial, coronal, and sagittal T1-weighted MRI of a 26-year-old female MS patient, superimposed with the $8_{LR} \times 10_{AP} \times 6_{IS} = 480$ cm^3 MRS VOI (*white outline*). **d-f** Corresponding slices in a 26-year-old healthy female control. Note the substantial, mostly (~75%) white matter, brain volume covered in this study and the extent of brain atrophy, reflected by enlarged lateral ventricles, subarachnoid spaces, and cortical sulci in the patient compared with her control

patients who suffer accelerated atrophy (compare Fig. 4a-c with Fig. 4d-f) [85], we summed all 640 Q_{ijk}s in each VOI and divided by its tissue volume (T_V), obtained from MRI segmentation [86]. This converted absolute amounts to an average concentration, suitable for cross-sectional comparison,

$$[i]_k = \frac{1}{T_V} \sum_{j=1}^{640} Q_{ijk} \approx \frac{0.033 \times V_V}{T_V \times S_R \times V_R} \times \sqrt{\frac{P_k^{180°}}{P_R^{180°}}} \times \sum_{j=1}^{640} S_{ijk} \quad \text{mol. i,} \tag{9}$$

Using 3D multi-voxel MRS to subsample and quantify many small voxels (Eq 8), and then synthesize from them one large VOI (Eq. 9), achieves two goals. First, it exploits the improved field homogeneity in the former. Second, it facilitates correction for local, small regions of field inhomogeneities, e.g., near air-tissue interfaces, on a voxel-by-voxel basis. Specifically, narrow, ~2 Hz, voxel metabolites' linewidths were conserved in their synthetic (aligned) sum, as shown in Fig. 5, whereas the *measured* linewidths from the 480-cm^3 VOI were 6±1 Hz. The improved spectral resolution facilitated more accurate peak-area quantification, especially for Cr and Cho.

Statistical Analyses

Levene's test was used to determine whether patients and controls exhibit different variability in either T_V or metabolite concentration, $[i]_k$, (i = NAA, Cr, or Cho). A Mann-Whitney test was used to compare patients and controls in terms of T_V and each $[i]_k$. Relations between [Cho] and [NAA] were investigated using the Spearman rank correlation test. Results are subsequently referred to as significant if at or above the 95% confidence level, i.e., $p \leq 0.05$.

Results

Each subject's average ^{1}H spectrum from the VOI, normalized to their T_V, is shown in Fig. 5. Individual T_Vs and average [NAA], [Cho], and [Cr] from Eq. (9), are compiled in Table 3 and compared, patients versus controls, in Fig. 6. [NAA] and T_V in the patients (median, mean ± standard deviation: 12.1, 12.1 ± 1.3 mM and 412.6, 410.8 ± 24.0 cm^3, respectively) were significantly lower than those in the controls (12.9, 13.2 ± 0.9 mM and 451.4, 447.7 ± 8.8 cm^3, respectively). In contrast, patients' median and mean [Cr] (6.7, 6.9 ± 0.8 mM) and [Cho] (2.0, 2.1 ± 0.2 mM) were significantly higher than the controls' (5.6, 5.6 ± 0.4 mM and 1.5, 1.6 ± 0.1 mM, respectively). The median and mean gray-matter volumes in the VOI (126, 131±16 cm^3 in the controls, 119, 117±8.6 cm^3 in the patients) exhibited a trend towards difference but without reaching statistical significance (p = 0.063).

Strong positive correlation (r = 0.76, p = 0.007) between [NAA] and [Cho] was found in the patient cohort but not amongst the controls. No significant correlation was found between the patients' EDSS scores and their T_V, [NAA], [Cr], or [Cho]. However, it should be noted that the sample size, the inherently ordinal nature of the EDSS scale, and the clustering of our patients' scores around 2.5, precluded adequate statistical power to discern such associations.

Two single-parameter metrics distinguished MS patients at 100% specificity

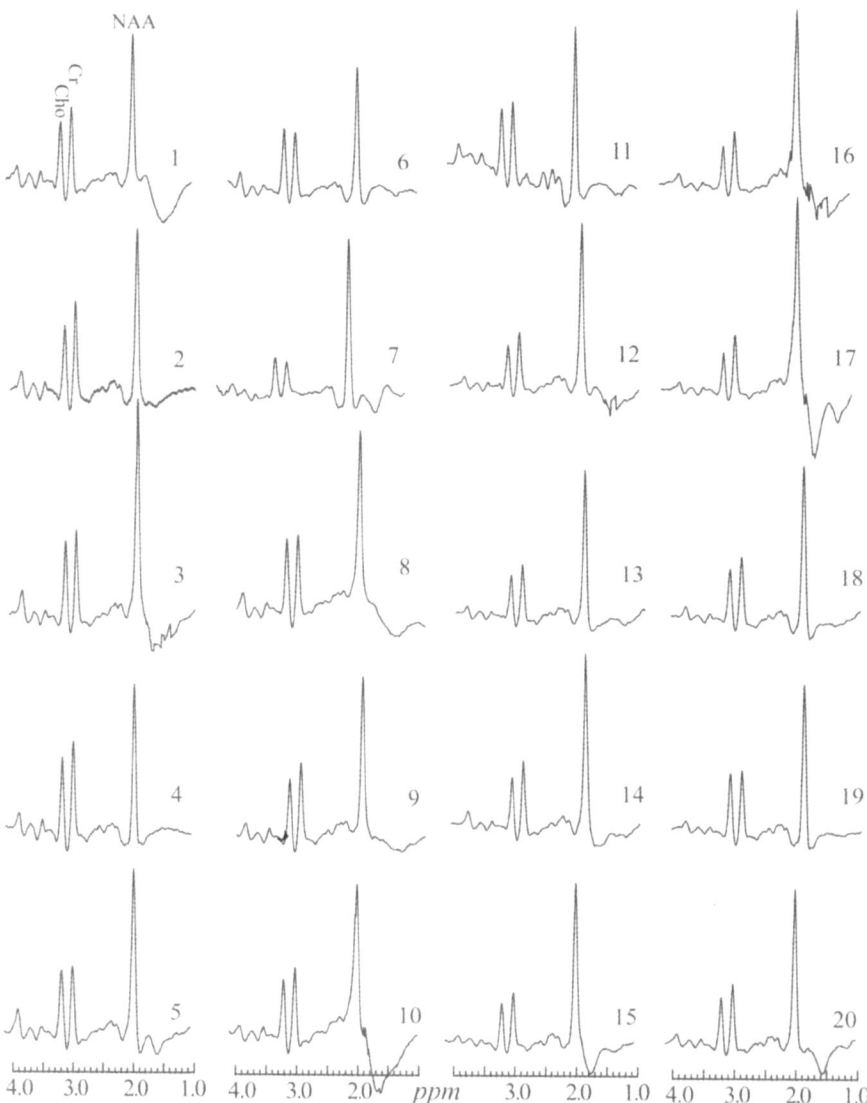

Fig. 5. Real part of the ¹H MR spectrum from the entire VOI corresponding to the patients (1-11) and controls (12-20) in Table 3. Each spectrum represents the sum of the localized ¹H-MRS contributions from all 640 voxels within the VOI, divided by its T_v. The spectra are on a common intensity (vertical) and indicated chemical shift (ppm) scales. Note the general characteristics of lower NAA and elevated Cho and Cr in the patients (spectra 1-11) compared with the controls (spectra 12-20)

Table 3. Demographic, clinical, volumetric, and metabolic details for the patients (1-11) and controls (12-20). Average T_V and $[i]_k$ (i=NAA, Cr and Cho) concentration differences in the 480 cm^3 VOI were statistically significant between the two cohorts (cf. Fig. 6)

Subject number	Age/ gender	Disease duration (years)	EDSS	T_V ± 24 cm^3	[NAA] ± 0.9 mM	[Cr] ± 0.4 mM	[Cho] ± 0.1 mM
1	26 F	5.9	1.5	385	11.7	7.5	2.1
2	31 F	7.9	3.5	403	10.7	6.7	1.7
3	32 F	7.0	1.5	447	13.4	6.7	2.1
4	36 F	6.9	2.5	368	12.1	8.1	2.3
5	37 F	5.0	0.0	434	14.0	7.3	2.3
6	42 M	6.9	0.0	423	10.8	5.7	2.0
7	43 F	6.9	3.5	427	10.5	5.7	1.8
8	43 M	3.9	3.5	388	14.1	7.7	2.5
9	44 F	6.9	2.0	403	12.1	6.7	1.9
10	47 M	7.9	6.0	413	10.8	6.8	2.0
11	48 F	10.9	2.5	429	12.9	6.7	2.0
12	21 F	–	–	454	14.5	5.5	1.5
13	21 F	–	–	451	12.9	5.2	1.4
14	25 F	–	–	458	13.2	6.1	1.6
15	26 F	–	–	456	12.1	5.0	1.4
16	30 M	–	–	453	12.2	5.6	1.5
17	36 F	–	–	440	14.1	5.4	1.3
18	36 F	–	–	436	14.4	6.3	1.7
19	39 M	–	–	453	12.5	5.6	1.8
20	48 F	–	–	434	12.7	6.0	1.7

and 91.9% sensitivity, correctly categorizing 19 of the 20 subjects: (1) [Cho] ≥ 1.8 mM, *higher* than its highest level amongst the controls (see Table 3 and Fig. 6); and (2) T_V ≤ 434 cm^3, lower than the smallest value in the controls cohort. Tests based on either [NAA] or [Cr] could not discriminate patients from controls with less than 10% error (sensitivities of 54.5% and 81.8%, respectively).

Discussion

Since atrophy is one of the apparent symptoms of early-stage MS [62, 85, 87] (compare Fig. 4a with Fig. 4b), we measured the T_V in the VOI in all subjects (see Table 3). The significant tissue loss observed in the patients compared with the controls (see Fig. 6a) was a reliable enough marker to differentiate the former from the latter at 100% sensitivity and greater than 90% specificity. However, while atrophy is the end point of all the processes that led to it, it is *nonspecific* as to what these were.

The sensitivity of MRI can be augmented with the specificity of ^{1}H-MRS focused on NAA [7, 70], present almost exclusively in neuronal cells [26] and considered a putative marker for their integrity and density [30, 31]. Therefore, its decrease in lesions and NAWM reflects either transient axonal impairment from inflammation and myelin breakdown, or permanent damage from loss of glial

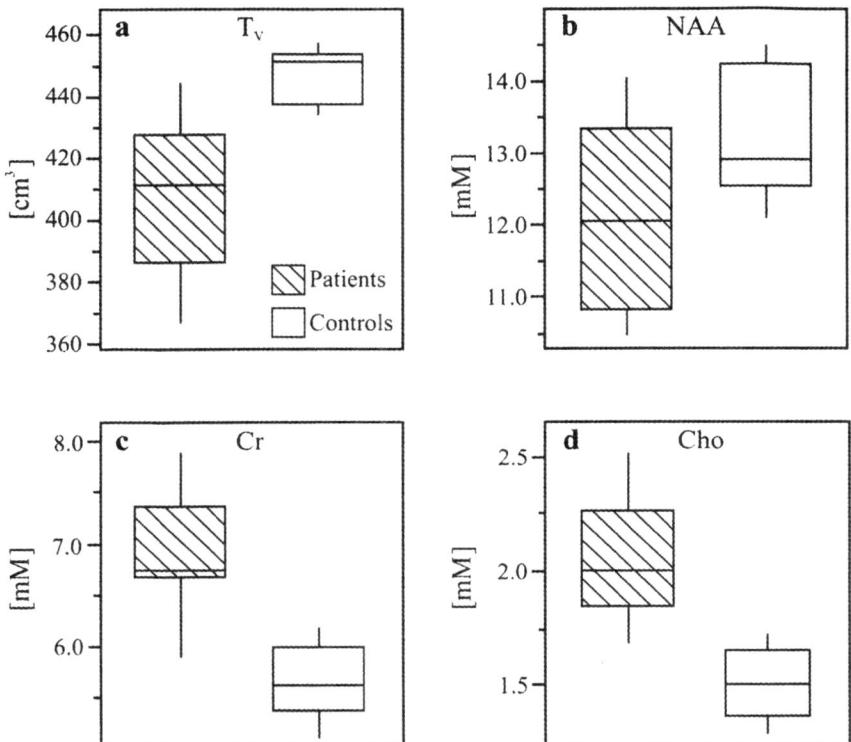

Fig. 6 a-d. Box plots displaying 25%, median and 75% (box), and ±95% (whiskers) range of the variation of the T_v, [NAA], [Cr], and [Cho] within the 480 cm3 MRS VOI for the RRMS patients and controls. Note the relative atrophy within the VOI in the patients (**a**) and the lower median NAA level (**b**) and higher levels of both Cr (**c**) and Cho (**d**) compared with the controls. All four differences were statistically significant

support, recurrent inflammation, and segmental demyelination [8, 18, 26, 30]. Indeed, consistent with previous reports, we observed significant [NAA] decline in patients versus controls (cf. Fig. 6b). Since it was normalized for T_v, we obtained both its loss to atrophy (average 9%) and concentration reduction in the remaining tissue (average 6%). However, while atrophy and NAA loss are complementary metrics of neuroaxonal damage, both are, unfortunately, end-stage phenomena.

This study represents two departures from the past paradigms. *First*, it employed 3D ^{1}H-MRS to examine substantial, 480-cm^3, VOIs (see Fig. 4) compared with the previous small, few to few tens of cubic centimeters, VOIs which left most of the NAWM invisible. *Second*, the metabolic focus was shifted to Cho- and Cr-containing compounds. The former, found in all cell membranes and considered indices of phospholipid metabolism [88], increase following inflammation and demyelination in lesions and NAWM in animals and humans [71, 89, 90]. The latter represent high-energy phosphates reserves in the cytosol of neurons and glial cells, providing for homeostasis and energy needs [91]. Its elevation has been attributed to synergetic effects of oligodendrocytic remyelination and astrocytic microgliosis in lesions [92], consistent with the notion that repair mechanisms are more efficient early on in MS.

We interpret the levels of and relationships between the metabolites to reflect NAWM *inflammation* (higher cellular density), *membrane turnover* (degradation/demyelination or synthesis/remyelination), and *gliosis* (astrocytic proliferation) in parallel, for the following four reasons:

1. Six percent reduction of [NAA], even after accounting for 9% atrophy in the VOI, probably indicates gliosis, i.e., replacement of axons by astrocytes.
2. Since significant astrocytosis often accompanies regions of axonal loss, if the observed [Cr] increase reflected only gliosis, inverse correlation with [NAA] would have been expected. Its absence indicates that [Cr] elevation also represents *re*-myelination.
3. Larger [Cho] and [Cr] variability in the patients than in the controls (cf. Figs. 6c and 6d), suggests pathological processes than are heterogeneous in age and histology. Therefore:
4. If [Cho] and [Cr] expressed the *same* process, *either* inflammation/demyelination, *or* remyelination, strong correlation between their levels would have been expected. Since such correlation was not found, these elevations must represent *parallel* independent processes, e.g., *de*- and *re*-myelination, consistent with MRS studies of NAWM [15, 16, 71-73, 93], as well as recent longitudinal biopsy findings of the evolution of new lesions, e.g., by Bitsch et al. [68].

Conclusions

Cho and Cr, individually, together, and in conjunction with the NAA, reflect an array of ongoing pathological processes widespread in the NAWM of MS patients, which persist even during the clinically quiescent phase(s) of the disease. Therefore, their noninvasive, in vivo assay in substantial regions could serve as specific surrogate markers for underlying pathological processes responsible for, and culminating in, the development of permanent axonal injury, reflected, ex post facto, by [NAA] decline. Since the accumulation of such injury could lead to irreversible disability, [Cho] and [Cr] might be earlier markers for the disease course/activity and therefore, perhaps, predict its response to anti-inflammatory/immunomodulatory therapy, definitive information that is unavailable from conventional imaging or MRI-based methods.

Acknowledgements. The authors are grateful to the study's patient coordinator Ms. Lois J. Mannon, R.T., and to our collaborators, Drs. Belinda S. Y. Li, David M. Moriarty, Matilde Inglese, Yulin Ge, Juan He, Andrew A. Maudsley, Brian J. Soher, James S. Babb, and Ms. J. Regal. This work was supported by NIH grants EB01015, NS37739, and NS29029.

References

1. Hauser SL (1994) Multiple sclerosis and other demyelinating diseases. In: Isselbacher KJ, Wilson JD, Martin JB, Fauci AS, Kasper DL (eds) Harrison's principles of internal medicine. McGraw-Hill, New York, pp 2287-2295
2. Weinshenker BG (1994) Natural history of multiple sclerosis. Ann Neurol 36:S6-S11
3. McFarland HF, Barkhof F, Antel J, Miller DH (2002) The role of MRI as a surrogate outcome measure in multiple sclerosis. Mult Scler 8:40-51
4. Filippi M (2001) Linking structural, metabolic and functional changes in multiple sclerosis. Eur J Neurol 8:291-297
5. Miki Y, Grossman RI, Udupa JK et al (1999) Differences between relapsing-remitting and chronic progressive multiple sclerosis as determined with quantitative MR imaging. Radiology 210:769-774
6. Allen IV, McKeown SR (1979) A histological, histochemical and biochemical study of the macroscopically normal white matter in multiple sclerosis. J Neurol Sci 41:81-91
7. Gonen O, Catalaa I, Babb JS et al (2000) Total brain N-acetylaspartate: a new measure of disease load in MS. Neurology 54:15-19
8. Arnold DL, De Stefano N, Narayanan S, Matthews PM (2001) Axonal injury and disability in multiple sclerosis: magnetic resonance spectroscopy as a measure of dynamic pathological change in white matter. In: Filippi M, Arnold D, Comi G (eds) Magnetic resonance spectroscopy in multiple sclerosis. Springer, Milan, pp 61-67
9. Miller DH, Grossman RI, Reingold SC, McFarland HF (1998) The role of magnetic resonance techniques in understanding and managing multiple sclerosis. Brain 121:3-24.
10. Filippi M, Inglese M, Rovaris M et al (2000) Magnetization transfer imaging to monitor the evolution of MS: a 1-year follow-up study. Neurology 55:940-946
11. Narayana PA, Doyle TJ, Lai D, Wolinsky JS (1998) Serial proton magnetic resonance spectroscopic imaging, contrast-enhanced magnetic resonance imaging, and quantitative lesion volumetry in multiple sclerosis. Ann Neurol 43:56-71
12. Filippi M, Rocca MA, Martino G et al (1998) Magnetization transfer changes in the normal appearing white matter precede the appearance of enhancing lesions in patients with multiple sclerosis. Ann Neurol 43:809-814
13. Rocca MA, Cercignani M, Iannucci G et al (2000) Weekly diffusion-weighted imaging of normal-appearing white matter in MS. Neurology 55:882-884
14. Loevner LA, Grossman RI, Cohen JA et al (1995) Microscopic disease in normal-appearing white matter on conventional MR images in patients with multiple sclerosis: assessment with magnetization-transfer measurements. Radiology 196:511-515
15. Davie CA, Barker GJ, Thompson AJ et al (1997) H-1 magnetic resonance spectroscopy of chronic cerebral white matter lesions and normal appearing white matter in multiple sclerosis. J Neurol Neurosurg Psychiatry 63:736-742
16. Fu L, Matthews PM, De Stefano N et al (1998) Imaging axonal damage of normal-appearing white matter in multiple sclerosis. Brain 121:103-113
17. Tortorella C, Viti B, Bozzali M et al (2000) A magnetization transfer histogram study of normal-appearing brain tissue in MS. Neurology 54:186-193
18. De Stefano N, Matthews PM, Fu LQ et al (1998) Axonal damage correlates with disability in patients with relapsing-remitting multiple sclerosis - results of a longitudinal magnetic resonance spectroscopy study. Brain 121:1469-1477
19. Nusbaum AO, Lu D, Tang CY, Atlas SW (2000) Quantitative diffusion measurements in focal multiple sclerosis lesions: correlations with appearance on TI-weighted MR images. AJR Am J Roentgenol 175:821-825
20. Rovaris M, Filippi M, Minicucci L et al (2000) Cortical/subcortical disease burden and cognitive impairment in patients with multiple sclerosis. AJNR Am J Neuroradiol 21:402-408

21. Ferguson B, Matyszak MK, Esiri MM, Perry VH (1997) Axonal damage in acute multiple sclerosis lesions. Brain 120:393-399
22. Lexa FJ, Grossman RI, Rosenquist AC (1994) MR of wallerian degeneration in the feline visual system: characterization by magnetization transfer rate with histopathologic correlation. AJNR Am J Neuroradiol 15:201-212
23. Narayanan S, Fu L, Pioro E et al (1997) Imaging of axonal damage in multiple sclerosis: Spatial distribution of magnetic resonance imaging lesions. Ann Neurol 41:385-391
24. De Stefano N, Narayanan S, Matthews PM et al (1999) In vivo evidence for axonal dysfunction remote from focal cerebral demyelination of the type seen in multiple sclerosis. Brain 122:1933-1939
25. Moffett JR, Namboodiri MA, Cangro CB, Neale JH (1991) Immunohistochemical localization of N-acetylaspartate in rat brain. Neuroreport 2:131-134
26. Simmons ML, Frondoza CG, Coyle JT (1991) Immunocytochemical localization of N-acetyl-aspartate with monoclonal antibodies. Neuroscience 45:37-45
27. Clark JB (1998) N-acetylaspartate: a marker for neuronal loss or mitochondrial dysfunction. Dev Neurosci 20:271-276
28. Davie CA, Hawkins CP, Barker GJ et al (1994) Serial proton magnetic resonance spectroscopy in acute multiple sclerosis lesions. Brain 117:49-58
29. De Stefano N, Narayanan S, Mortilla M et al (2000) Imaging axonal damage in multiple sclerosis by means of MR spectroscopy. Neurol Sci 21:S883-887
30. Trapp BD, Peterson J, Ransohoff RM et al (1998) Axonal transection in the lesions of multiple sclerosis. N Engl J Med 338:278-285
31. Bjartmar C, Kidd G, Mork S et al (2000) Neurological disability correlates with spinal cord axonal loss and reduced N-acetyl aspartate in chronic multiple sclerosis patients. Ann Neurol 48:893-901
32. Matthews PM, Arnold DL (2001) Magnetic resonance imaging of multiple sclerosis: new insights linking pathology to clinical evolution. Curr Opin Neurol 14:279-287
33. Gonen O, Grossman RI (2001) New magnetic resonance spectroscopy strategies. In: Filippi M, Arnold D, Comi G (eds) Magnetic resonance spectroscopy in multiple sclerosis. Springer, Milan, pp 97-112
34. Gonen O, Viswanathan AK, Catalaa I et al (1998) Total brain N-acetylaspartate concentration in normal, age-grouped females: quantitation with non-echo proton NMR spectroscopy. Magn Reson Med 40:684-689
35. Sadovnick AD (2001) To treat or not to treat the person with clinical multiple sclerosis - a dilemma. Neurol Sci 22:205-207
36. Schwid SR, Bever CT (2001) The cost of delaying treatment in multiple sclerosis. What is lost is not regained. Neurology 56:1620
37. Comi G, Filippi M, Barkhof F et al (2001) Effect of early interferon treatment on conversion to definite multiple sclerosis: a randomised study. Lancet 357:1576-1582
38. Goodkin DE (2000) Interferon beta-1b in secondary progressive MS: clinical and MRI results of a 3-year randomized controlled trial. Neurology 54:6
39. Jacobs LD, Cookfair DL, Rudick RA et al (1996) Intramuscular interferon beta-1 alpha for disease progression in relapsing multiple sclerosis. Ann Neurol 39:285-294
40. Johnson KP, Brooks BR, Cohen JA et al (1995) Copolymer-1 reduces relapse rate and improves disability in relapsing-remitting multiple sclerosis - results of a phase-III multicenter, double-blind, placebo-controlled trial. Neurology 45:1268-1276
41. Compston A (1999) Interferon beta in multiple sclerosis - Reply. Lancet 354:512-513
42. NIH (1993) Multiple sclerosis. National Institutes of Health, Bethesda, Md, pp 8-11. (NIH Guide)
43. Hartung HP (2000) NICE and drugs for multiple sclerosis. Lancet 356:1114-1114
44. Willoughby E, Paty D (1998) Scales for rating impariment in multiple sclerosis: a critique. Neurology 38:1793-1798

45. Filippi M, Iannucci G, Tortorella C et al (1999) Comparison of MS clinical phenotypes using conventional and magnetization transfer MRI. Neurology 52:588-594
46. Krupp LB, Elkins LE (2000) Fatigue and declines in cognitive functioning in multiple sclerosis. Neurology 55:934-939
47. Tas MW, Barkhol F, van Walderveen MAA, Polman CH et al (1995) The effect of gadolinium on the sensitivity and specificity of MR in the initial diagnosis of multiple sclerosis. AJNR Am J Neuroradiol 16:259-264
48. Jacobs LD, Kaba SE, Miller CM et al (1997) Correlation of clinical, magnetic resonance imaging, and cerebrospinal fluid findings in optic neuritis. Ann Neurol 41:392-398
49. Fazekas F, Barkhof F, Filippi M et al (1999) The contribution of magnetic resonance imaging to the diagnosis of multiple sclerosis. Neurology 53:448-456
50. Filippi M, Horsfield MA, Tofts PS et al (1995) Quantitative assessment of MRI lesion load in monitoring the evolution of multiple sclerosis. Brain 118:1601-1612
51. Udupa JK, Samarasekera S (1996) Fuzzy connectedness and object definition: theory, algorithms, and applications in image segmentation. Graph Models Image Process 58:246-261
52. Ge Y, Grossman RI, Udupa JK et al (1999) Longitudinal quantitative analysis of brain atrophy in relapsing-remitting and secondary-progressive multiple sclerosis. Radiology 214:665-670
53. De Stefano N, Matthews PM, Antel JP et al (1995) Chemical pathology of acute demyelinating lesions and its correlation with disability. Ann Neurology 38:901-909
54. De Stefano N, Narayanan S, Francis GS et al (2001) Evidence of axonal damage in the early stages of multiple sclerosis and its relevance to disability. Arch Neurol 58:65-70
55. Arnold DL, Riess GT, Matthews PM et al (1994) Use of proton magnetic resonance spectroscopy for monitoring disease progression in multiple sclerosis. Ann Neurol 36:76-82
56. Taylor DL, Davis SE, Obrenovitch TP et al (1995) Investigation into the role of N-acetylaspartate in cerebral osmoregulation. J Neurochem 65:275-281
57. Ebers GC, Yee IM, Sadovnick AD, Duquette P (2000) Conjugal multiple sclerosis: population-based prevalence and recurrence risks in offspring. Canadian Collaborative Study Group. Ann Neurol 48:927-931
58. Sadovnick AD, Yee IM, Ebers GC (2000) Factors influencing sib risks for multiple sclerosis. Clin Genet 58:431-435
59. Dyment DA, Willer CJ, Scott B et al (2001) Genetic susceptibility to MS: a second stage analysis in Canadian MS families. Neurogenetics 3:145-151
60. Dyment DA, Cader MZ, Willer CJ et al (2002) A multigenerational family with multiple sclerosis. Brain 125:1474-1482
61. Fox NC, Miller DH, Thompson AJ (2000) Progressive cerebral atrophy in MS: a serial study using registered, volumetric MRI - reply. Neurology 55:1243-1243
62. Rudick RA, Fisher E, Lee JC et al (1999) Use of the brain parenchymal fraction to measure whole brain atrophy in relapsing-remitting MS. Neurology 53:1698-1704
63. Scott TF, Schramke CJ, Novero J, Chieffe C (2000) Short-term prognosis in early relapsing-remitting multiple sclerosis. Neurology 55:689-693
64. Rogatko A, Litwin S (1996) Phase II studies: which is worse, false positive or false negative? J Natl Cancer Inst 88:462
65. Sormani MP, Miller DH, Comi G et al (2001) Clinical trials of multiple sclerosis monitored with enhanced MRI: new sample size calculations based on large data sets. J Neurol Neurosurg Psychiatry 70:494-499
66. Duquette P, Despault L, Knobler RL et al (1995) Interferon beta-1b in the treatment of multiple sclerosis - final outcome of the randomized controlled trial. Neurology 45:1277-1285
67. Forbes RB, Lees A, Waugh N, Swingler RJ (1999) Population based cost utility study of interferon beta-1b in secondary progressive multiple sclerosis. Br Med J 319:1529-1533

68. Bitsch A, Bruhn H, Vougioukas V et al (1999) Inflammatory CNS demyelination: histopathologic correlation with in vivo quantitative proton MR spectroscopy. AJNR Am J Neuroradiol 20:1619-1627
69. Arnold DL, Matthews PM, Francis G, Antel J (1990) Proton magnetic resonance spectroscopy of human brain in vivo in the evaluations of multiple sclerosis: assessment of the load of disease. Magn Reson Med 14:154-159
70. Arnold DL, De Stefano N, Matthews PM, Trapp BD (2001) N-acetylaspartate: usefulness as an indicator of viable neuronal tissue. Ann Neurol 50:823; discussion 824-825
71. Husted CA, Goodin DS, Hugg JW et al (1994) Biochemical alterations in multiple sclerosis lesions and normal-appearing white matter detected by in vivo 31P and 1H spectroscopic imaging. Ann Neurol 36:157-165
72. Tourbah A, Stievenart JL, Iba-Zizen MT et al (1996) In vivo localized proton NMR spectroscopy of normal appearing white matter in patients with multiple sclerosis. J Neuroradiol 23:49-55
73. Rooney WD, Goodkin DE, Schuff N et al (1997) 1H MRSI of normal appearing white matter in multiple sclerosis. Mult Scler 3:231-237
74. Sarchielli P, Presciutti O, Pelliccioli GP et al (1999) Absolute quantification of brain metabolites by proton magnetic resonance spectroscopy in normal-appearing white matter of multiple sclerosis patients. Brain 122:513-521
75. Suhy J, Rooney WD, Goodkin DE et al (2000) H-1 MRSI comparison of white matter and lesions in primary progressive and relapsing-remitting MS. Mult Scler 6:148-155
76. Urenjak J, Williams SR, Gadian DG, Noble M (1993) Proton nuclear magnetic resonance spectroscopy unambiguously identifies different neural cell types. J Neurosci 13:981-989
77. Gonen O, Murdoch JB, Stoyanova R, Goelman G (1998) 3D multivoxel proton spectroscopy of human brain using a hybrid of 8th-order Hadamard encoding with 2D-chemical shift imaging. Magn Reson Med 39:34-40
78. Lublin FD, Reingold SC (1996) Defining the clinical course of multiple sclerosis: results of an international survey. National Multiple Sclerosis Society (USA) Advisory Committee on Clinical Trials of New Agents in Multiple Sclerosis. Neurology 46:907-911
79. Kurtzke JF (1983) Rating neurologic impairment in multiple sclerosis: an expanded disability status scale (EDSS). Neurology 33:1444-1452
80. Hu J, Javaid T, Arias-Mendoza F et al (1995) A fast, reliable, automatic shimming procedure using 1H chemical-shift-imaging spectroscopy. J Magn Reson B 108:213-219
81. Soher BJ, Young K, Govindaraju V, Maudsley AA (1998) Automated spectral analysis III: application to in vivo proton MR spectroscopy and spectroscopic imaging. Magn Reson Med 40:822-831
82. Soher BJ, van Zijl PCM, Duyn JH, Barker PB (1996) Quantitative proton MR spectroscopic imaging of the human brain. Magn Reson Med 35:356-363
83. Christiansen P, Tofts P, Larsson HB et al (1993) The concentration of N-acetyl aspartate, creatine + phosphocreatine, and choline in different parts of the brain in adulthood and senium. Magn Reson Imaging 11:799-806
84. Duyn JH, Gillen J, Sobering G et al (1993) Multisection proton MR spectroscopic imaging of the brain. Radiology 188:277-282
85. Ge Y, Grossman RI, Udupa JK et al (2001) Brain atrophy in relapsing-remitting multiple sclerosis: fractional volumetric analysis of gray matter and white matter. Radiology 220:606-610
86. Hutchinson M, Rusinek H, Nenov VI et al (1997) Segmentation analysis in functional MRI: activation sensitivity and gray-matter specificity of RARE and FLASH. J Magn Reson Imaging 7:361-364
87. Fox NC, Jenkins R, Leary SM et al (2000) Progressive cerebral atrophy in MS - a serial study using registered, volumetric MRI. Neurology 54:807-812
88. McIlwain H, Bachelard H (1985) Biochemistry and central nervous system. Churchill Livingstone, Edinburgh, pp 282-335

89. Arnold DL, Matthews PM, Francis GS et al (1992) Proton magnetic resonance spectroscopic imaging for metabolic characterization of demyelinating plaques. Ann Neurol 31:235-241

90. Brenner RE, Munro PMG, Williams SCR et al (1993) The proton NMR spectrum in acute EAE: the significance of the change in the Cho:Cr ratio. Magn Reson Med 29:737-745

91. Miller BL (1991) A review of chemical issues in 1H NMR spectroscopy: N-acetyl-L-aspartate, creatine and choline. NMR Biomed 4:47-52

92. Mader I, Roser W, Kappos L et al (2000) Serial proton MR spectroscopy of contrast-enhancing multiple sclerosis plaques: absolute metabolic values over 2 years during a clinical pharmacological study. AJNR Am J Neuroradiol 21:1220-1227

93. Pan JW, Hetherington HP, Vaughan JT et al (1996) Evaluation of multiple sclerosis by 1H spectroscopy imaging at 4.1 T. Magn Reson Med 36:72-77

Chapter 5

Perfusion MRI

W. Rashid, D.H. Miller

Introduction

Perfusion is a measure of blood supply to a tissue. The term is used to describe the volume of blood passing through an organ normalised to the mass of the organ. It is an important indicator of tissue health and viability as it offers an insight into the efficiency of delivery of nutrients and removal of waste products, and is measured in millilitres of blood per gram of tissue per unit time. As the brain receives a significant proportion of total circulation – around 20% – it follows that changes in cerebral blood flow (CBF) may play an important role in disease pathogenesis and monitoring.

Magnetic resonance imaging (MRI) is the most sensitive imaging tool available to visualise the anatomy of the brain in vivo. The availability of this investigation has improved our understanding of pathology in a number of diseases of the central nervous system, not least with the discovery of high-signal-intensity white matter lesions in T2-weighted imaging in multiple sclerosis (MS) [1]. As MRI techniques have evolved, an increasing number of parameters can now be determined, among them the measurement of functional and metabolic variables. One of these new opportunities is the evaluation of cerebral perfusion, which can be achieved by calculating the concentration of a magnetised tracer agent in the target area of interest.

A number of disease processes may be revealed by estimating CBF. In studies of cerebral infarction, perfusion imaging with an additional diffusion sequence can be used to identify an ischaemic penumbra which is potentially useful in guiding thrombolytic therapy [2]. In addition to this, assessments of patients with dementia reveal regional cerebral blood volume deficits [3], indicating sensitivity to neurodegeneration. Conversely, conditions involving activation or inflammation have shown a focus or increase in perfusion, as shown in studies investigating epilepsy [4] and in the evaluation of HIV [5]. This shows the great versatility of this measurement in the elucidation of pathological processes.

Although the diagnosis of MS has been improved through the use of MRI [6], the correlation of lesion load seen on T2-weighted images with clinical parameters [7] is modest. Quantitative studies with magnetisation transfer ratio (MTR) [8] and diffusion-weighted imaging (DWI) [9] have revealed abnormality in areas outside visible lesions, but with only marginally improved clinical correlations. The measurement of perfusion has the potential to provide further insight into the presence and nature of disease processes in MS and to improve concordance between imaging parameters and clinical scales. This chapter provides an overview of perfusion MRI techniques and summarises the observations that have been made when investigating diseases of the central nervous system, with a particular emphasis on MS. A detailed explanation of the modelling of the measurements is, however, beyond the scope of this review.

Perfusion Imaging Techniques

Non-MRI Techniques

The first accurate measure of cerebral perfusion was reported in 1945 by Kety [10,11]. The method used the inhalation of an inert tracer, nitrous oxide, and quantification was based on the Fick principle [12], equating the quantity of oxygen taken up by the brain to the product of blood flow through the brain, and the difference in the arterial and venous oxygen concentration. The advent of radionucleotide methods, single photon emission tomography (SPECT) and positron emission tomography (PET) have seen an increasing interest in the evaluation of CBF in healthy volunteers and in patients with varying conditions, including MS [13]. Both techniques have reasonable reproducibility (PET 12% whole brain [14] and SPECT 11% hemisphere [15]), but they are invasive in that they require administration of radionucleotide agents and in general have poorer spatial and anatomical resolution than MRI techniques, especially SPECT.

MRI Techniques

These techniques use either exogenous tracer agents, such as paramagnetic contrast substances, or endogenous molecules, for instance, labelled arterial water. Perfusion is calculated from the serial measurement of tracer concentration as it passes through the the organ being analysed. In principle, these techniques have several advantages over their rivals, not least the ability to register images to high-resolution structural sequences, allowing more accurate CBF evaluation in normal-appearing brain tissue and lesions. In addition, the use of radioactive material is avoided. Two different classes of MRI methods exist based on the type of tracer employed.

Exogenous Contrast Techniques

A paramagnetic substance, such as gadolinium (Gd), is used in this analysis. The modelling assumes the tracer is wholly intravascular, and dynamic imaging (high-speed acquisition following a rapid injection of contrast) or steady-state estimation (measurement after equilibrium concentration is reached in blood) is undertaken. The latter is rarely used because it has a less favourable signal-to-noise ratio (SNR) and can only measure cerebral blood volume, not CBF. With dynamic methods the T2 (spin-echo) or T2* (gradient-echo) signal loss, due to the intravascular bolus of Gd travelling through the capillaries, can be used to generate a concentration-time curve of Gd in the imaging area [16]. From this, the relative values of CBF, cerebral blood volume and mean transit time (MTT) can be calculated [16]. The measures are not quantitative but are compared those of to a "normal" area. Absolute values can be obtained by measuring the arterial input function, but this is prone to error in its evaluation.

An advantage of this technique is that it has better spatial resolution than does endogenous tracer modelling, thus allowing smaller regions of interest (ROIs), e.g. MS lesions, to be analysed. A better SNR can also be achieved, improving the sensitivity of the technique. The measurement relies on the perfusion being constant and unaffected by the tracer. Also, it is assumed in the modelling, which is based on tracer kinetics [17-19], that the contrast agent is well mixed with the blood and that its concentration is accurately measured. One possible source of error is the delay between Gd injection and image acquisition, which potentially allows dispersal of the agent before the concentration is measured, leading to underestimation of CBF. High-speed bolus injection is required in order to produce a "tight" bolus, which will increase SNR and avoid recirculation problems. Brain coverage can be limited due to the need for fast image acquisition to accurately characterise the signal curve as the tracer passes quickly through the tissue. Further difficulties arise from the assumption that the tracer remains intravascular. If there is any loss of integrity in the blood-brain barrier (BBB), for example, as has been demonstrated in MS [20], this may lead to leakage of contrast, causing an increase in T1 effects and leading to an underestimation of perfusion. Also, the contributions of tracer in large, non-perfusing vessels can cause an overestimation of true tissue perfusion. The need to inject a contrast agent is a further limitation of this approach.

Endogenous Contrast Techniques

This mode of imaging uses magnetic labelled arterial water as an endogenous contrast agent. The signal change caused by the reduced longitudinal magnetisation of the tracer can be used to measure perfusion. Inversion usually takes place in a proximal labelling plane, with image acquisition undertaken by a high-speed EPI sequence after a delay in which the labelled blood is able to enter the region of interest. Two sets of images are collected, one with inversion and the other without, so on subtraction the signal from the labelled blood remains with the static tissue signal removed. Standard, single-compartment modelling assumes free permeability of the capillary wall to water. The process is termed arterial spin labelling (ASL) and has two subtypes, pulsed (PASL) and continuous (CASL), which terms describe the manner in which inversion takes place. Both sequences permit quantitative values and are dependent on the T1 relaxation time of arterial blood, the labelling efficiency, tissue T1 relaxation and the transit time for blood to travel between the inversion plane and the tissue [21].

Pulsed methods use a short RF pulse to label a relatively large volume of spins. The technique is easier to implement but suffers from a lower SNR than CASL. A number of different methods have been developed, the first being EPISTAR (echo planar imaging and signal targeting with alternating radiofrequency) [22] and its commonly used variation, FAIR (flow-sensitive alternating inversion recovery) [23].

CASL uses continuous RF inversion in a plane perpendicular to a major feeding artery in a distal imaging region. As blood crosses the inversion plane, its longitudinal magnetisation is inverted, causing a loss of signal in the images, dependent on blood perfusion. Using a control sequence with no net labelling, this reduction can be measured and a perfusion map can be generated [21]. A consequence of the way inversion is achieved are magnetisation transfer (MT) effects in the static tissue of the image slice, which can shorten the T1 relaxation time of water in the extravascular space. A control sequence with matching MT effects [24] removes any contribution from this in the perfusion map. Some of the SNR advantage in comparison to PASL is lost because the blood takes longer to travel to the tissue from the more distant labelling site used with CASL. Modifications to the modelling have removed the assumption of free permeability of the capillary wall to water, which has been shown to cause errors in perfusion quantification [25]. Results on a cohort of healthy controls appear promising, with a good whole-brain perfusion reproducibility of 8% [26].

ASL is becoming increasingly employed as a research tool of particular interest in functional imaging. In addition, when there is disruption to the BBB it may be a more appropriate method than using intravascular contrast modelling with exogenous techniques. It does, however, suffer from inherently lower SNR and spatial resolution, which make it a less suitable technique in certain clinical applications.

Clinical Applications of Perfusion MRI

As the sophistication and accuracy of MRI methods improve, the clinical and research potential of perfusion MRI increases.

Cerebrovascular Disease

This group of disorders occur as a direct result of abnormality in CBF. It therefore follows that the measurement of CBF has the potential to be extremely informative both in defining pathophysiology and in guiding management. Most studies have used exogenous contrast methods of MRI, chiefly because of the better spatial resolution and SNR profile. Using perfision MRI in combination with DWI, an ischaemic penumbra of "at-risk" tissue can be identified as an area of normal diffusion and decreased perfusion [2]. With DWI alone, only infarcted tissue is visualised (as reduced diffusion acutely, then later on as increased diffusion). Encouraging clinical correlation has been reported between the extent of this salvageable tissue area and the presence of long-term disability [27]. Given the increasing use of thrombolytic therapy in acute stroke and the inherent risks of such agents, the identification of patients who may benefit most from intervention would be very useful, emphasising the potential future importance of this form of imaging.

The versatility of perfusion measurement is also shown by its ability to reveal changes in chronic cerebrovascular conditions involving vascular insufficiency in an arterial territory, such as the common carotid, after the infusion of acetazolamide. This has traditionally been done using PET and, most commonly, SPECT, but evaluations using Gd-bolus MRI have recently been reported [28, 29] to show perfusion changes following the administration of the agent.

Degenerative Disorders

Studies have particularly evaluated Alzheimer's disease and frontotemporal dementia [3]. As perfusion is thought to reflect tissue health and metabolism, perfusion measurement may offer a further insight into these disorders, which often exhibit normal structural imaging apart from the development of global or regional atrophy. Both MRI methods have been used to investigate dementia [30, 31], and typical estimations have shown a regional decrease in blood volume corresponding to neural reductions. Whether this alteration is secondary to this loss or is involved in the pathological process that instigates it has yet to be determined.

Cerebral Tumours

The character of capillary blood flow to neoplasms in the brain may reflect its pathological grading, with higher-graded tumours often acquiring large collateral circulations [32]. Perfusion has been used to measure flow around tumours in order to clarify their nature and also guide stereotactic biopsy [33, 34]. Because CBF to an area of radiation necrosis has a different pattern, the technique can be used to distinguish a suspicious region seen on structural imaging from tumour recurrence following radiotherapy [35]. Gd bolus methods are again preferred because of resolution and SNR considerations. Because of its better visualisation of small vessels, T2 SE methods may be preferable to T2* weighted modelling [36].

Epilepsy

Certain refractory seizure types may be amenable to surgery if a suitable resectable focus can be identified. Previous SPECT analysis has shown a correlation between increased rCBF in a focal area and EEG in status epilepticus [4]. ASL modelling has been reported to show mesial temporal hypoperfusion in relation to seizure focus [37].

Clinical Research and Functional Studies

ASL has become an increasingly attractive technique in research studies, chiefly because of its ability to measure perfusion quantitatively, giving better inter- and intra-subject comparability in longitudinal studies. In contrast to Gd bolus MRI, the values are not calculated in relation to a "normal area", making ASL potentially more reliable in conditions where diffuse pathology is likely. Another benefit of absolute quantification is in the role of functional studies. BOLD (blood oxygenation level-dependent) effects have been the parameter estimated in activation studies, but, potentially, perfusion values have more accuracy as they do not include venous circulation effects which can be a source of error [38].

Multiple Sclerosis

Initially PET and SPECT techniques were used, with Brookes et al. [13] in 1984 offering the first insight into perfusion changes in MS. Other studies have since been undertaken measuring either blood flow or glucose uptake as a marker of tissue metabolism. All studies report regional decreases in grey matter areas, with two studies observing lower CBF in areas of white matter [39-41]. The most common regions of grey matter hypoperfusion were seen in frontal and temporal areas [13, 39-41], with one study noting greater changes in the left hemisphere [42].

Three Gd bolus studies have been reported investigating MS. The largest was undertaken by Haselhorst et al. [43] who investigated 25 subjects (17 with relapsing-remitting, 7 with secondary progressive and 1 with primary progressive disease) and found a decrease in relative CBF in frontal lobe grey matter. Evaluation of lesions showed an increase in acute, enhancing plaques and hypoperfusion in chronic T1-hypointense lesions. This could indicate an inflammatory process in acute plaques (with increased metabolism and hence perfusion) and degenerative pathological change in other ROIs (with decreased metabolism and perfusion), demonstrating the complex nature of MS. Jensen et al. [44] also reported perfusion changes in visible lesions in 7 patients. However, they observed a decrease in CBV might in all types, unlike Haselhorst et al. [43]. They hypothesised that oedema in active inflammatory lesions be causing this difference. Petrella et al. [45] also showed similar findings to Jensen et al. [44] in 9 patients, and suggested that interstitial oedema from BBB breakdown and perivascular inflammation was causing small-vessel compression, thereby decreasing capillary capacity.

Although Gd bolus MRI has been used for the reasons stated earlier, it does have some disadvantages. A major source of inaccuracy is the assumption that the exogenous contrast agent remains intravascular. In a condition like MS where disruption of BBB has been shown to occur [20], this is particularly relevant. In addition, only relative values are calculated in relation to a "normal" area, often the thalamus. Studies with other MRI modalities have shown diffuse changes in both grey and white matter in MS, including the thalamus [46-49], which further confounds the perfusion value measured. Further modelling improvements to ASL, for example the addition of a two-compartment solution modelling for the selective permeable nature of the BBB [25], mean that endogenous techniques should be more accurate. A recent report using CASL with these modifications showed for the first time an increase in white matter perfusion in relapsing-remitting and secondary progressive MS [50]. Further preliminary work has shown a decrease in perfusion in regions of the cortex and deep grey matter in progressive forms of MS, consistent with a neurodegenerative process. This may offer an insight into the nature of the pathology in different subtypes of the disease and appears to be a promising tool for further studies in MS.

Conclusions

The increasing sophistication of MRI and the new techniques this tool has yielded have provided new insights into pathological processes in many diseases. MS is a condition with complex and heterogeneous pathological features, and with pathogenetic mechanisms that are not well elucidated. These new techniques are of value in providing an opportunity to improve our understanding and thereby develop more effective therapies.

Perfusion methodologies are constantly evolving and interest in their use in clinical and research applications is growing, e.g. in the evaluation of the extent of stroke. Because perfusion changes show sensitivity to different disease processes, the technique has definite potential in the monitoring and investigation of MS.

Acknowledgements. The authors particularly wish to thank Laura M. Parkes for her advice and comments and the Multiple Sclerosis Society of Great Britain and Northern Ireland for their continuing support of the NMR Research Unit.

References

1. Jacobs L, Kinkel W, Polanchini I, Kinkel R (1986) Correlations of nuclear magnetic resonance imaging, computerised tomography and clinical profiles in multiple sclerosis. Neurology 36:27-34
2. Sorensen AG, Buonanno FS, Gonzalez RG et al. (1996) Hyperacute stroke: evaluation with combined multisection diffusion-weighted and haemodynamically weighted echo-planar MR imaging. Radiology 199:391-401
3. Detre JA, Alsop DC (1999) Perfusion magnetic resonance imaging with continuous arterial spin labelling: methods and clinical applications in the central nervous system. Eur J Radiol 30:115-124
4. Warach S, Levin JM, Schomer D et al (1994) Hyperperfusion of ictal seizure focus demonstrated by magnetic resonance perfusion imaging: SPECT, EEG and clinical correlation. AJNR Am J Neuroradiol 15:965-968
5. Chang L, Ernst T, Leonido-Yee M, Speck O (2000) Perfusion MRI detects rCBF abnormalities in early stages of HIV-cognitive motor complex. Neurology 54:386-396
6. McDonald WI, Compston A, Edan G et al (2001) Recommended diagnostic criteria for multiple sclerosis: guidelines from the international panel on the diagnosis of multiple sclerosis. Ann Neurol 50:121-127
7. Kurtzke JF (1983) Rating neurological impairment in multiple sclerosis; an expanded disability status scale (EDSS). Neurology 33:1444-1452
8. Filippi M, Campi A, Dousset V et al (1995) A magnetisation transfer imaging study of normal appearing white matter in multiple sclerosis. Neurology 45:478-482
9. Christiansen P, Gideon P, Thomsen C et al (1993) Increased water self diffusion in

chronic plaques and in apparently normal white matter in patients with multiple sclerosis. Acta Neurol Scand 87:195-199

10. Kety SS, Schmidt CF (1945) The determination of cerebral blood flow in man by the use of nitrous oxide in low concentrations. Am J Physiol 143:53

11. Kety SS (1996) The cerebral circulation. In: Fishman AP, Richards DW (eds) Circulation of the blood: men and ideas. Oxford University Press, New York

12. Fick A (1870) Ueber die Messung des Blutquantums in den Herzventrikeln. Sitzungsber Phys Med Ges, Würzburg, 9 July 1870

13. Brooks DJ, Leenders KL, Head G et al (1984) Studies on regional cerebral oxygen utilisation and cognitive function in multiple sclerosis. J Neurol Neurosurg Psychiatry 47:1182-1191

14. Matthew E, Andreason P, Carson RE et al (1993) Reproducibility of resting cerebral blood flow measurements with $H_2^{15}O$ positron emission tomography in humans. J Cereb Blood Flow Metab 13:748-754

15. Podreka I, Baumgartner C, Suess E et al (1989) Quantification of regional cerebral blood flow with IMP-SPECT. Reproducibility and clinical relevance of flow values. Stroke 20:183-191

16. Rosen BR, Belliveau JW, Vevea JM, Brady TJ (1990) Perfusion imaging with NMR contrast agents. Magn Reson Med 14:249-265

17. Zierler KL (1962) Theoretical basis of indicator-dilution methods for measuring flow and volume. Circ Res 10:393-407

18. Zierler KL (1965) Equations for measuring blood flow by external monitoring of radioisotopes. Circ Res 16:309-321

19. Axel L (1980) Cerebral blood flow determination by rapid-sequence computed tomography. Radiology 137:676-686

20. Tofts PS, Kermode AG (1989) Blood-brain barrier permeability in multiple sclerosis using labelled DTPA with PET, CT and MRI. J Neurol Neurosurg Psychiatry 52:1019-1020

21. Detre JA, Leigh JS, Williams DS, Koretsky AP (1992) Perfusion imaging. Magn Reson Med 23:37-45

22. Edelman RR, Siewert B, Darby DG et al (1994) Qualitative mapping of cerebral blood flow and functional localisation with echo-planar MR imaging and signal targeting with alternating radio frequency. Radiology 192:513-520

23. Kwong KK, Belliveau JW, Chesler DA et al (1992) Dynamic magnetic resonance imaging of human brain activity during primary sensory stimulation. Proc Natl Acad Sci USA 89:5675-5679

24. Alsop DC, Detre JA (1998) Multisection cerebral blood flow MR imaging with continuous arterial spin labelling. Radiology 208:410-416

25. Parkes LM, Tofts PS (2002) Improved accuracy of human cerebral blood perfusion measurements using arterial spin labelling. Accounting for capillary water permeability. Magn Reson Med 48:27-41

26. Parkes LM, Rashid W, Chard DT, Tofts PS (2002) Normal cerebral perfusion measurements using CASL: reproducibility, age and gender effects. Proc of the 10th Annual Meeting Int Soc Magn Reson Med, Hawaii, p 431

27. Tievsky AL, Gonzalez RG, Lev MH et al (1998) Correlation of DWI/MTT mismatch and MRA/CTA in acute stroke. In: Proceedings of the 36th Annual Meeting of the American Society of Neuroradiology, Philadelphia

28. Guckel FJ, Brix G, Schmiedek P et al (1996) Cerebrovascular reserve capacity in patients with occlusive cerebrovascular disease: assessment with dynamic susceptibility contrast-enhanced MR imaging and the acetazolamide stimulation test. Radiology 201:405-412

29. Tanaka C, Fukunaga M, Ebisu T et al (1997) Cerebral perfusion imaging using FAIR: acetazolamide effects and clinical application. Fifth Scientific Meeting and Exhibition of the Society of Magnetic Resonance in Medicine, Vancouver, p 579

30. Renshaw P, English C, Satlin A et al (1996) Comparison of brain SPECT and dynamic susceptibility contrast MR imaging in Alzheimer's disease. In: Proceedings of the 82nd Scientific Assembly and Annual Meeting of the Radiological Society of North America, Chicago, p 131

31. Alsop DC, Detre JA, Grossman M (2000) Assessment of cerebral blood flow in Alzheimer's disease by spin-labelled magnetic resonance imaging. Ann Neurol 47:93-100

32. Brem S, Cotran R, Folkman J (1972) Tumor angiogenesis: a quantitative method for histologic grading. J Natl Cancer Inst 48:347-356

33. Aronen H, Gazit IE, Louis DN et al (1994) Cerebral blood volume maps of gliomas: comparison with tumor grade and histologic findings. Radiology 191:41-51

34. Knopp EA, Cha S, Johnson G et al (1999) Glial neoplasms: dynamic contrast-enhanced T2*-weighted MR imaging. Radiology 211:791-798

35. Lev MH, Schaefer PW, Barest GD et al (1997) Radiation necrosis or glioma recurrence? Magnetic resonance relative cerebral blood volume imaging in proton beam patients. In: Proceedings of the 82nd Scientific Assembly and Annual Meeting of the Radiological Society of North America, Chicago

36. Fisel CR, Ackermann JL, Buxton RB et al (1991) MR contrast due to microscopically heterogeneous magnetic susceptibility: numerical simulations and applications to cerebral physiology. Magn Reson Med. 17:336-347.

37. Wolf RL, Alsop DC, French JA et al (2001) Detection of mesial temporal lobe hypoperfusion in patients with temporal lobe epilepsy using arterial spin labelled perfusion MRI. AJNR Am J Neuroradiol 22:1334-41

38. Detre JA, Wang J (2002) Technical aspects and utility of fMRI using BOLD and ASL. Clin Neurophysiol 113:621-634

39. Lycke J, Wikkelsö C, Bergh A et al (1993) Regional cerebral blood flow in multiple sclerosis measured by single photon emission tomography with technetium-99m hexamethyl-propyleneamine oxime. Eur Neurol 33:163-167

40. Bakshi R, Miletich RS, Kinkel PR et al (1998) High-resolution fluordeoxyglucose positron emission tomography shows both global and regional cerebral hypometabolism in multiple sclerosis. J Neuroimaging 8:228-234

41. Blinkenberg M, Rune K, Jensen CV et al (2000) Cortical cerebral metabolism correlates with MRI lesion load and cognitive dysfunction in MS. Neurology 54:558-564

42. Signorini M, Paulesu E, Friston K et al (1999) Rapid assessment of regional cerebral metabolic abnormalities in single subjects with quantitative and nonquantitative [18F]FDG PET: a clinical validation of statistical parametric mapping. Neuroimage 9:63-80

43. Haselhorst R, Kappos L, Bilecen D et al (2000) Dynamic susceptibility contrast MR imaging of plaque development in multiple sclerosis: application of an extended blood-brain barrier leakage correction. J Magn Reson Imaging 11:495-505

44. Jensen CV, Rostrup E, Blinkenberg M et al (1995) Relative regional cerebral blood-volume in MS. Proc Soc Magn Reson 2:1297

45. Petrella JR, Yang Y, Richert N et al (1997) Dynamic contrast MR measurements of relative cerebral blood volume in enhancing multiple sclerosis lesions: Comparison to nonenhancing lesions and normal appearing white matter. Proc Intern Soc Magn Reson Med 1:646

46. Bakshi R, Benedict RH, Bermel RA et al (2002) T2 hypointensity in the deep gray matter of patients with multiple sclerosis: a quantitative magnetic resonance imaging study. Arch Neurol 59:62-68

47. Filippi M, Bozzali M, Comi G (2001) Magnetisation transfer and diffusion tensor MR imaging of basal ganglia from patients with multiple sclerosis. J Neurol Sci 183:69-72

48. Wylezinska M, Cifelli A, Matthews P et al (2002) Neuronal damage in thalamic grey matter in relapsing-remitting multiple sclerosis. Proc Int Soc Magn Reson Med 10:592

49. Wylezinska M, Cifelli A, Matthews P, Jezzard P (2001) Thalamic neuronal loss in multiple sclerosis: a combined structural and spectroscopic study. Proc Int Soc Magn Reson Med 9:473
50. Rashid W, Parkes LM, Ingle GT et al (2002) Comparative investigation of cerebral perfusion in multiple sclerosis using a novel technique. Proc Int Soc Magn Reson Med 10:1264

Chapter 6

Functional MRI

M. Filippi, M.A. Rocca

Introduction

Multiple sclerosis (MS) is a chronic inflammatory disease of the central nervous system (CNS) characterized by a proteiform pattern of clinical manifestations and a highly variable evolution. During the past decade, significant efforts have been devoted to improving our understanding of the pathophysiology of MS, with the ultimate goal of identifying and monitoring treatment strategies that have the potential to modify the evolution of the disease positively.

The classical notion that MS is a demyelinating disease affecting the white matter of the CNS has been challenged by the demonstration that: (1) axonal pathology in macroscopic brain lesions and in the normal-appearing brain tissue (NABT) is an important feature of the disease from its earliest phases [1-5]; (2) gray matter is not spared by the disease, as shown by pathologic [6-8] and in vivo quantitative magnetic resonance imaging (MRI) studies [9-12]; and (3) brain plasticity may help to explain recovery and the maintenance of a normal level of function in the presence of irreversible tissue loss. In case of axonal loss, the factors that traditionally have been viewed as potentially able to limit the clinical impact of MS pathology [13-15], including resolution of acute inflammation, remyelination, and redistribution of voltage-gated sodium channels in persistently demyelinated axons, are all likely to have a very limited role, if any. Brain plasticity is a well-known feature of the human brain that is likely to have several pathologic substrates, including increased axonal expression of sodium channels [16], synaptic changes, increased recruitment of parallel existing pathways or "latent" connections, and reorganization of distant sites, and it may have a major adaptive role in limiting the functional consequences of axonal loss. In this chapter, we summarize the main functional MRI (fMRI) studies performed in patients with MS, highlighting how they are changing our views on the ability of the brain in MS to limit the clinical consequences of irreversible structural tissue damage.

Basic Principles of fMRI

FMRI is a relatively new technique that is being widely used to study the neuronal mechanisms of CNS functioning, since it is inexpensive, noninvasive, safe, and

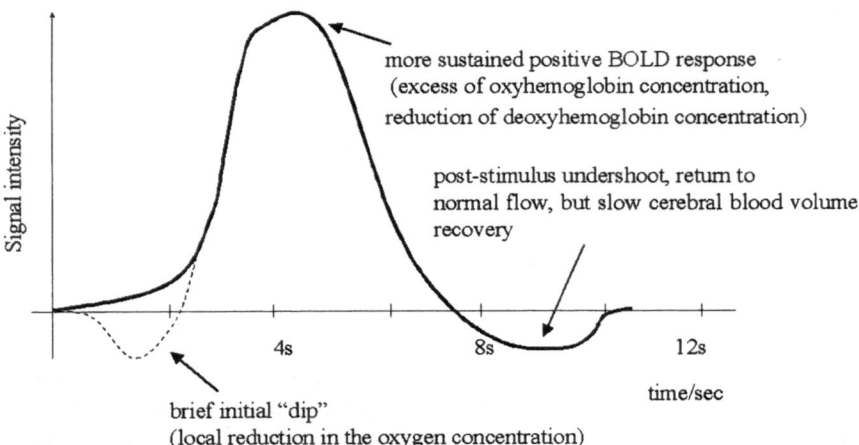

more sustained positive BOLD response
(excess of oxyhemoglobin concentration,
reduction of deoxyhemoglobin concentration)

post-stimulus undershoot, return to
normal flow, but slow cerebral blood volume
recovery

brief initial "dip"
(local reduction in the oxygen concentration)

Fig. 1. Course of the blood-oxygenation-level-dependent (BOLD) response to an increase in neuronal activity. The *dotted line* indicates a brief initial dip of the BOLD response that has not been proved definitively. (Reproduced from [19], with permission)

gives a higher spatial resolution than other functional imaging techniques such as positron emission tomography.

The signal changes seen during fMRI studies depend on the blood-oxygena-tion-level-dependent (BOLD) mechanism, which in turn involves changes of the transverse magnetization relaxation time – either T2*, in a gradient echo sequence, or T2, in a spin echo sequence [17]. Activation of cerebral tissue causes an increase in local synaptic activity, which results in a rise in blood flow and oxygen consumption. The increase in blood flow is greater than the oxygen consumption, giving rise to an increase in the ratio between oxygenated and deoxygenated hemoglobin, which enhances the MRI signal [17-19] (Fig. 1). As these signal changes are very modest (usually ranging from 0.5% to 1.5%), it is necessary to obtain a large amount of brain images acquired during alternating periods of activation (motor, sensory, and cognitive) and rest [20]. By analyzing these data with appropriate statistical methods, it is possible to obtain information about the location and the extent of specific areas involved in the performance of a given task in healthy subjects and in patients [21, 22].

fMRI in MS

fMRI is being widely used for the study of MS, for several reasons. First, the strength of the correlation between clinical and MRI findings is still limited, despite the availability of other modern quantitative MR techniques with increased specificity to the heterogeneous substrates of MS [23-28]. Secondly, definition of the nature and timing of cortical adaptive mechanisms could be critical in establishing a prognosis. And, thirdly, it could be useful to evaluate the effect of therapeutic strategies specifically targeted to enhance these adaptive functional changes of the cortex.

The main problem in the interpretation of the results of fMRI studies is that the observed changes may be biased by differences in task performance between patients and controls. Clearly, this is a major issue in MS, a disease which typically causes impairment of various functional systems, and this has limited the overall value of the earlier fMRI studies of patients with MS [29, 30].

Nevertheless, this limitation has been elegantly overcome by many recent fMRI studies of MS, which have investigated the brain patterns of activations in MS patients with different disease courses and with different levels of clinical disability.

fMRI in Patients with Clinically Isolated Syndromes (CIS) Suggestive of MS

The first manifestation of MS is in many cases an acute, remitting, clinically isolated syndrome (CIS) involving the optic nerves, brain stem, or spinal cord [31]. Recent quantitative MRI studies have shown that irreversible tissue loss can occur in these patients [32-34] as well as in those with an early form of relapsing-remitting (RR) MS [2, 34-37], despite the absence or paucity of clinical manifestations outside of the acute phases. To investigate how early cortical reorganization occurs in the course of MS, fMRI has been used to study the visual and motor systems of patients with CIS suggestive of MS [38-40].

A preliminary study of the visual system [37] conducted on patients who had recovered from a single episode of acute unilateral optic neuritis (ON) demonstrated that, while in controls visual stimulation activated only the primary visual cortex, extensive activations of the claustrum, lateral temporal and posterior parietal cortices, and thalamus in addition to the activation of the primary visual cortex were found in patients when the clinically affected eye was studied. Stimulation of the clinically unaffected eye resulted in activation of only the visual cortex and the right insula claustrum. In addition, the volume of the extraoccipital activation in patients with ON was found to correlate strongly with the latency of the visual evoked potentials. Since all the activated extraoccipital areas have been shown to be part of a complex network responsible for multimodal integration [41], the results of this study fit with the notion that a functional reorganization of the cortex might represent an adaptive response to a persistently abnormal visual input.

Recently, fMRI has also been used to study, within 3 months from first clinical relapse, movement-associated cortical activations in patients at presentation with CIS highly suggestive of MS following a simple motor task with the dominant hand [39]. The relationship between the extent of cortical activation and the extent of overall brain axonal pathology, measured using an unlocalized magnetic resonance spectroscopy (MRS) technique, was also investigated [39]. Compared with healthy controls, CIS patients had a different pattern of movement-associated cortical activations, which was mainly characterized by increased activation of

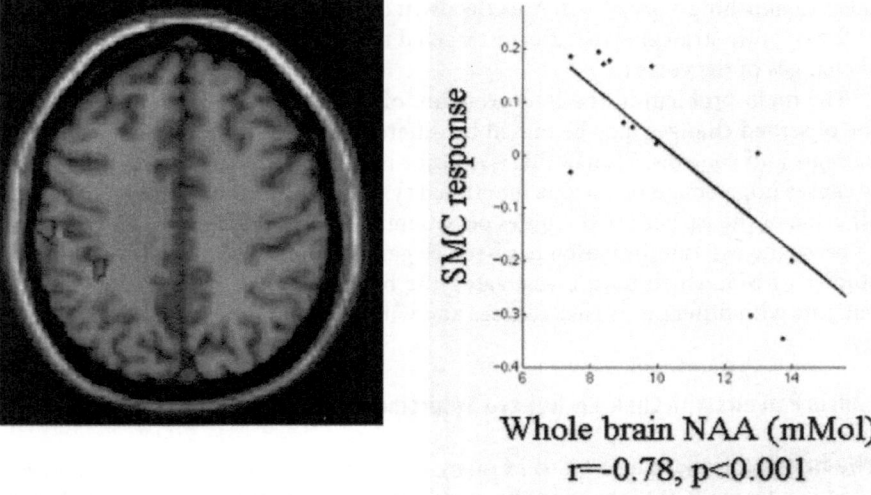

Whole brain NAA (mMol)
r=-0.78, p<0.001

Fig. 2. A Relative contralateral primary sensorimotor cortex activation in patients at presentation with clinically isolated syndromes suggestive of multiple sclerosis during the performance of a simple motor task with the right hand, in comparison to healthy volunteers. The scatterplot of the correlation between the relative activation of the contralateral primary sensorimotor cortex and whole brain *N*-acetylaspartate concentrations is also shown **(B)**

the contralateral primary sensorimotor cortex (SMC) (Fig. 2). In comparison with healthy volunteers, CIS patients also had a significantly reduced whole brain *N*-acetylaspartate (WBNAA) concentration. Interestingly, a strong correlation was found between the extent of the activation of the contralateral primary SMC and the reduction of WBNAA concentration (Fig. 2). This suggests that functional cortical reorganization might contribute to the maintenance of normal functional capacities from the earliest stage of MS.

Recently, Pantano et al. [40] studied a group of ten patients with early MS diagnosed according to the McDonald criteria [42] and with a previous episode of hemiparesis. During the performance of a simple motor task with the right hand, they found that, in comparison with healthy volunteers, patients had increased activation of several cortical areas, mainly located in the ipsilateral hemisphere. The extent of the activations was correlated with disease duration. The discrepant results obtained by these two fMRI studies of patients with CIS [39, 40] are probably due to differing clinical characteristics of the patients recruited (for instance, the mean disease duration in the study of Pantano et al. [40] was of 24.3 months, versus a mean of 34 days in that by Filippi et al. [39]). In addition, the fact that the patients included in the study of Pantano et al. [40] had had a previous hemiparesis does not allow the interference of altered task performance on the results to be completely ruled out, as is the case for the other study [39].

fMRI During Recovery from an Acute Relapse

Two different studies [29, 43], used fMRI to monitor cortical changes during recovery from an acute relapse in patients with RRMS. In the study by Clanet et al. [29], two patients were evaluated serially during recovery from an acute paralysis of the upper limbs. In one of these patients, who was initially unable to perform the task, no activation was observed at baseline. However, when the "normal" hand was used to perform the task, the primary SMC was activated bilaterally. During clinical recovery of the affected hand, a bilateral activation of the primary SMC with a transient significant increase of the activated area was observed. These findings have been confirmed and extended by a subsequent study of Reddy et al. [43], who used serial MRS and fMRI exams ination to follow a patient after the onset of acute hemiparesis, who had a new large demyelinating lesion in the corticospinal tract. They showed that clinical recovery preceded complete normalization of NAA and was accompanied by relative increases of ipsilateral primary SMC and supplementary motor area (SMA) activations. This finding suggests that this altered pattern of recruitment of elements of the cortical motor network might have contributed to the restoration of normal functioning despite the injury to the corticospinal tract. The correlation of MRS and fMRI findings also confirms that dynamic reorganization of the motor cortex can occur in response to an axonal injury associated with MS relapses.

fMRI in Patients with RRMS without Clinical Disability

Recent postmortem [4, 5] and in-vivo quantitative MR [26, 32-34, 44] studies have shown that irreversible axonal damage is a major component of the pathology of RRMS. Despite this, quite a large number of patients with RRMS, at least during a certain period of the disease course, experience relapses and accumulation of MRI lesion burden without being left with any major residual neurologic deficits.

To understand better whether adaptive cortical reorganization has a role in limiting the impact of irreversible tissue loss in these patients, a recent study has investigated the brain patterns of cortical activations during the performance of a simple motor task in 14 nondisabled RRMS patients [45]. In this study, the magnitude of the correlation between fMRI changes and the extent of T2-visible lesions, as well as the severity of MS pathology in lesions and NABT, measured using magnetization transfer (MT) and diffusion tensor (DT) MRI, were also investigated. Compared to healthy controls, MS patients showed increased activations of the contralateral primary SMC, the SMA bilaterally, the cingulate motor area bilaterally, the contralateral ascending bank of the sylvian fissure (SII), and the contralateral intraparietal sulcus. Strong correlations were found between the extent of fMRI activations and several MT and DT MRI metrics of structural brain damage (Fig. 3). This study demonstrated that cortical activation occurs over a rather distributed sensorimotor network in nondisabled RRMS patients and gave additional evidence that increased recruitment of this cortical network contributes to limiting the functional impact of MS damage associated with

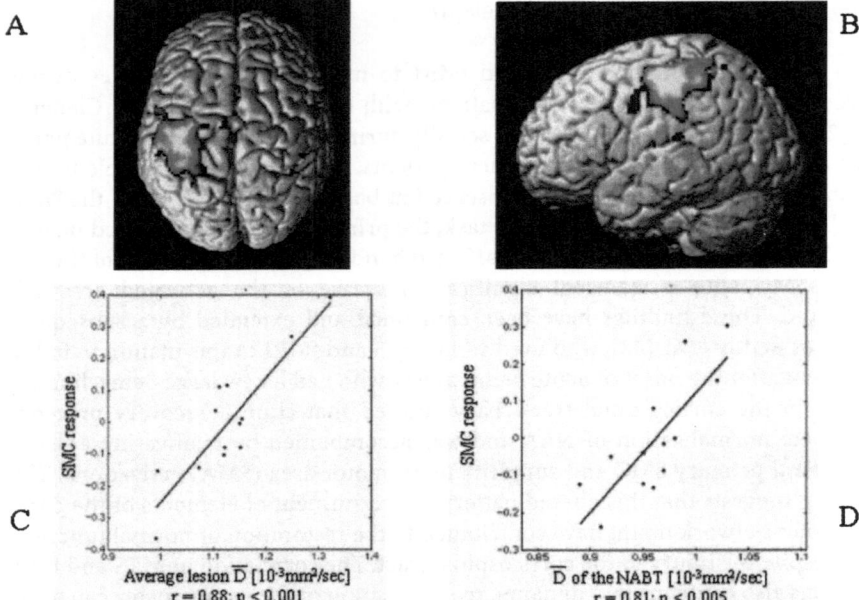

Fig. 3 A, B. Brain patterns of cortical activations on a rendered brain in nondisabled relapsing-remitting MS patients during the performance of a simple motor task with their right hand. Widespread activation of several areas of the sensorimotor network (including the contralateral primary and secondary sensorimotor cortex, the supplementary motor area, and the ipsilateral postcentral gyrus) is visible. The scatterplots of the correlations between the relative activation of the contralateral primary sensorimotor cortex and average lesion mean diffusivity (C) and mean diffusivity of the normal-appearing brain tissue (D) are also shown. (Reproduced from [45], with permission)

macroscopic lesions and subtle NABT changes. Interestingly, in another group of patients [46] with clinical characteristics similar to those of patients recruited in the previous study [45], but who complained of fatigue, a reduced activation of a complex movement-associated cortical/subcortical network, including the cerebellum, the rolandic operculum, the thalamus, and the middle frontal gyrus, was demonstrated in comparison with matched nonfatigued MS patients [46] (Fig. 4). A strong correlation between the reduction of thalamic activity and the severity of fatigue was also found (Fig. 4). This suggests that a less marked cortical recruitment might be associated to the appearance of clinical symptoms in MS.

fMRI in Patients with RRMS and Secondary Progressive MS and Mild to Moderate Clinical Disability

Several studies have been performed to investigate the visual and motor system in patients with MS and mild to moderate clinical disability.

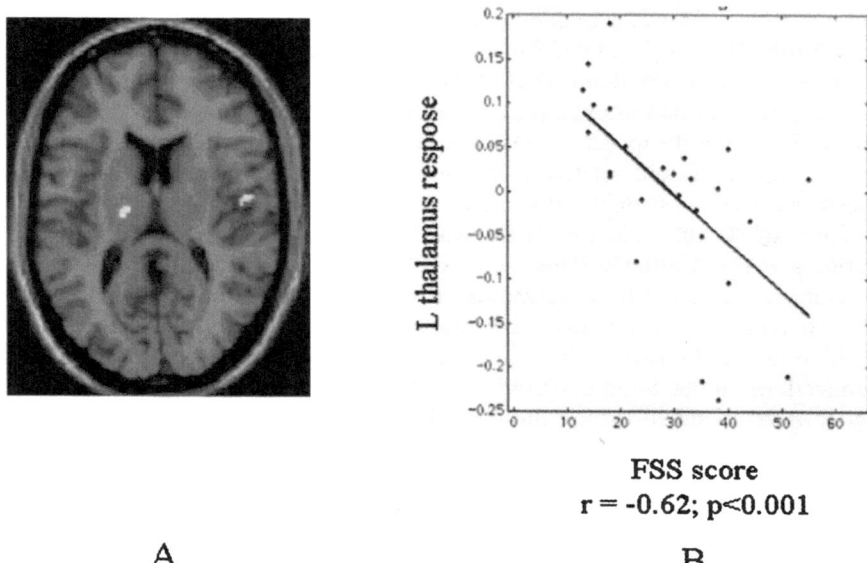

FSS score
r = -0.62; p<0.001

A   B

Fig. 4. A Relative cortical activations in right-handed nonfatigued MS patients of the contralateral thalamus and ipsilateral rolandic operculum during the performance of a simple motor task in comparison with right-handed fatigued MS patients performing the same task. The scatterplot of the correlation between the relative activation of the contralateral thalamus and fatigue severity scale score in the whole sample of MS patients is also shown (**B**). (Reproduced from [46], with permission)

A preliminary study interrogated the visual system [47] and showed that MS patients with unilateral ON had a smaller activation of the visual cortex after stimulation of the affected and unaffected eyes when compared to healthy subjects. On average, patients with optimal recovery from the ON showed increased visual cortex activation compared with those with poor or no recovery. A more recent study [48] performed in nine patients with previous ON confirmed the results of the previous study [47] and showed that ON patients not only have reduced activation of the primary visual cortex, but also a reduced fMRI percentage signal change in this region, again suggesting an abnormality of its synaptic input.

Movement-associated brain activations have been investigated in patients with RRMS and secondary progressive (SP) MS with mild to moderate clinical disability. Lee et al. [30] used fMRI to characterize the site and the volume of SMC and SMA activations during flexion-extension of the last four fingers of the right hand in 12 clinically stable patients and found increased SMA activation in MS patients compared with controls, reduced recruitment of the contralateral SMC in patients with more severe functional impairment than those with milder impairment, and, in the whole patient sample, increased ipsilateral SMC activation with increasing lesion load in the contralateral hemisphere. They also found a posterior shift of the center of activation of the contralateral SMC in patients compared to controls. The magnitude of the SMC posterior shift increased with increasing T2-visible lesion loads. Reddy et al. [49] obtained MRS and fMRI scans from nine MS patients who had unimpaired motor or sensory hand function. They found that activation of the ipsilateral SMC with simple hand movements was increased by a mean of fivefold relative to normal controls and that the extent of this increase correlated strongly with decreasing levels of brain NAA.

Since subtle abnormalities of the NABT are an additional feature of RRMS patients [9-11, 44, 50], the impact of NABT damage, assessed using DT MRI, on movement-associated fMRI activations in patients with RRMS and nonspecific abnormalities on T2-weighted conventional MRI of the brain was investigated [51]. To assess the role of the nondominant hemisphere and interhemispheric connections on the dominant hand movement-associated pattern of activations, patients were studied during the performance of simple motor tasks with the dominant and the nondominant hand, and the results obtained from the two tasks combined. Compared to healthy volunteers, during the performance of a simple motor task with their dominant hand, MS patients showed increased activation of several areas of the sensorimotor network, including the ipsilateral SMA (Fig. 5), the ipsilateral superior frontal sulcus, and the contralateral thalamus. The increased recruitment of the SMA correlated with the peak height and position of the mean diffusivity histogram of the normal-appearing gray matter (Fig. 5). By contrast, compared to MS patients, healthy subjects showed increased activation of the ipsilateral primary SMC. When the performance of the two tasks (with the

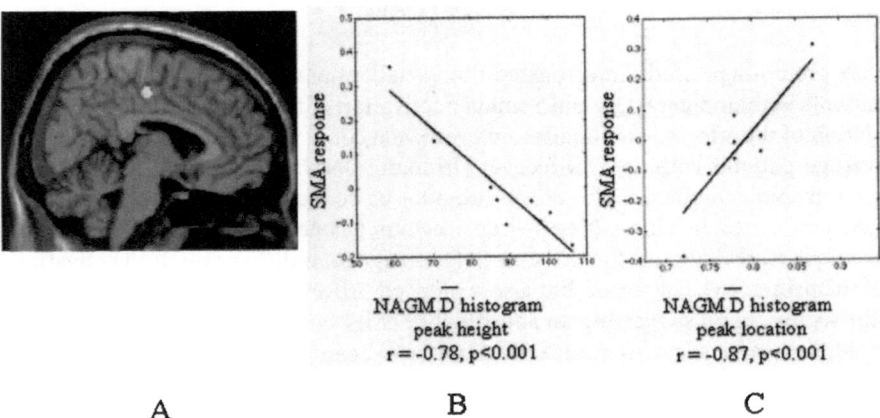

NAGM D histogram
peak height
r = -0.78, p<0.001

NAGM D histogram
peak location
r = -0.87, p<0.001

A   B   C

Fig. 5. A Relative cortical activation of the ipsilateral supplementary motor area in patients with clinically definite MS and nonspecific brain MRI findings during the performance of a simple motor task with their clinically unimpaired and fully normally functioning right hand in comparison to matched healthy volunteers. The scatterplots of the correlations between the relative activation of the supplementary motor area and mean diffusivity histogram peak height (**B**) and location (**C**) of the normal-appearing gray matter are also shown

dominant and the nondominant hand) were combined, MS patients showed increased activation of the SMA and reduced activation of the ipsilateral SMC. These findings might be explained by enhanced "transcallosal inhibition," a mechanism that is well known to occur in humans and has been postulated to be responsible for the control of homologous hand muscle during unilateral movements [52]. The central role of the corpus callosum in interhemispheric connectivity has been underpinned by a recent study [53] that measured low-frequency BOLD fluctuations to demonstrate reduced functional connectivity between the right and the left hemisphere primary motor cortices in MS patients.

Recent preliminary work has shown that the pattern of movement-associated cortical activations is determined by both the extent of brain injury and disability [54]. Cortical activations during a simple motor task have been studied in three groups of SPMS patients classified as follows: group 1: no clinical impairment and normal "axonal equivalents"; group 2: no clinical impairment and 20% reduction in "axonal equivalents"; and group 3: 40% reduction in the movement performance of the hand and 20% reduction in "axonal equivalents." The "injury contrast" (i.e., group 2 vs. group 1) showed increased activation of the SMA and premotor cortex in patients of group 2, whereas the "impairment contrast" (i.e., group 3 vs. group 2) showed increased activation of the SMC and of the parietal cortex, bilaterally in group 3.

Increased recruitment of several cortical areas of patients with RRMS and mild clinical disability has also been shown during the performance of a simple cognitive task. Staffen et al. [55] compared the brain pattern of activations of 21 MS patients with that of a group of sex- and age- matched healthy volunteers during the performance of the Paced Visual Serial Addition Task (PVSAT). MS patients, who showed no difference in task performance compared to healthy subjects, had increased activation of several regions located in the frontal and parietal lobes. This different pattern of activation, accompanied with intact task performance, suggests once again the compensatory role of brain plasticity in MS.

fMRI in Patients with Primary Progressive Multiple Sclerosis

Patients with primary progressive (PP) MS represent 10%-15% of patients with MS and are characterized by the progressive accumulation of disability from the onset of the disease [56]. This is in contrast with the small amount of lesions visible on conventional MRI scans of the brain and cord [57-60]. However, MT and DT MRI as well as MRS studies have shown diffuse changes in the NABT of the brain and cervical cord of these patients, which have been found to be correlated with disability accumulation [24, 34, 44, 61-63]. Work with DT MRI has also detected widespread cortical gray matter pathology in these patients [11].

Understanding the extent to which cortical reorganization occurs in PPMS and whether it has an adaptive role might be rewarding in terms of a better understanding of the pathophysiology of progressive disability in MS and in terms of planning treatment strategies for these patients. At present, only two studies [64, 65] have investigated the role of cortical plasticity in limiting the functional consequences of widespread tissue damage in patients with PPMS. In one study [64], the patterns of brain activations following simple and complex motor tasks were assessed in 30 right-handed patients with PPMS and variable degrees of motor impairment and compared with those from 15 right-handed sex- and age-matched controls. Significant cortical activation changes during both the simple and the complex motor tasks were found in PPMS patients, who showed different patterns of cortical activations with varying degrees of clinical impairment. During the performance of a simple motor task with the clinically unaffected limbs (Fig. 6), PPMS patients had more significant activations of the contralateral SMA, the upper bank of the sylvian fissure (SII) bilaterally, and several regions of the frontal (bilateral middle frontal gyrus and contralateral inferior frontal gyrus) and temporal (ipsilateral insula and bilateral superior temporal gyrus) lobes than did healthy volunteers. These findings indicate a marked cortical reorganization taking place in brain regions involved in different phases of movement planning and execution. Interestingly, the observed pattern of cortical activations involved a widespread network usually considered to function in motor, sensory, and multimodal integration processing [41]. This is consistent with the notion that, in humans, motor planning and execution is based on a distributed, interacting cortical network which extends well beyond "classical" motor areas [41]. During the performance of a simple task with an affected limb, PPMS patients showed increased activations of the ipsilateral cingulate motor area (CMA) and the ipsilateral postcentral gyrus. Since CMA activation in healthy subjects has been related to learning of new motor tasks and is also thought to reflect task difficulty [66-68], a possible explanation for the increased CMA recruitment found in PPMS patients might be that the patients tended to perceive the simple experimental task as a sort of novel task, which consequently needed to be "re-learned." Finally, during the execution of a more complex task, PPMS patients showed increased activations of the ipsilateral thalamus, the middle frontal gyrus bilaterally, and several other sensory regions, including an ipsilateral area located in the visual cortex. Visual-sensory interactions are known to occur in humans [68], and, again, they might be enhanced in PPMS patients in an attempt to compensate for the functional impairment due to subcortical white matter damage.

In the second study [65], the extent of brain activations during simple hand movements was correlated to lesion burden as seen on T2-weighted MRI scans, and to MT ratio (MTR) and average mean diffusivity ($\bar{D}$) of brain T2-visible lesions, NABT, and cervical cord from 26 PPMS patients with fully normal motor function in their right upper limbs. T2-visible lesion volume reflects the extent of overall MS macroscopic pathology, whereas MTR and $\bar{D}$ also provide quantitative information about tissue integrity at the microscopic level. A low MTR indicates reduced exchange of magnetization between the protons in the brain tissue and the surrounding water protons, and in a postmortem study [70] it was found to be strongly associated with the degree of myelin and axon loss. $\bar{D}$ is a measure of the average water molecular motion independent of any tissue directionality and is affected by cellular size and integrity [71]. The hypothesis tested was that if cortical adaptive responses have the potential to limit the accumulation of disability

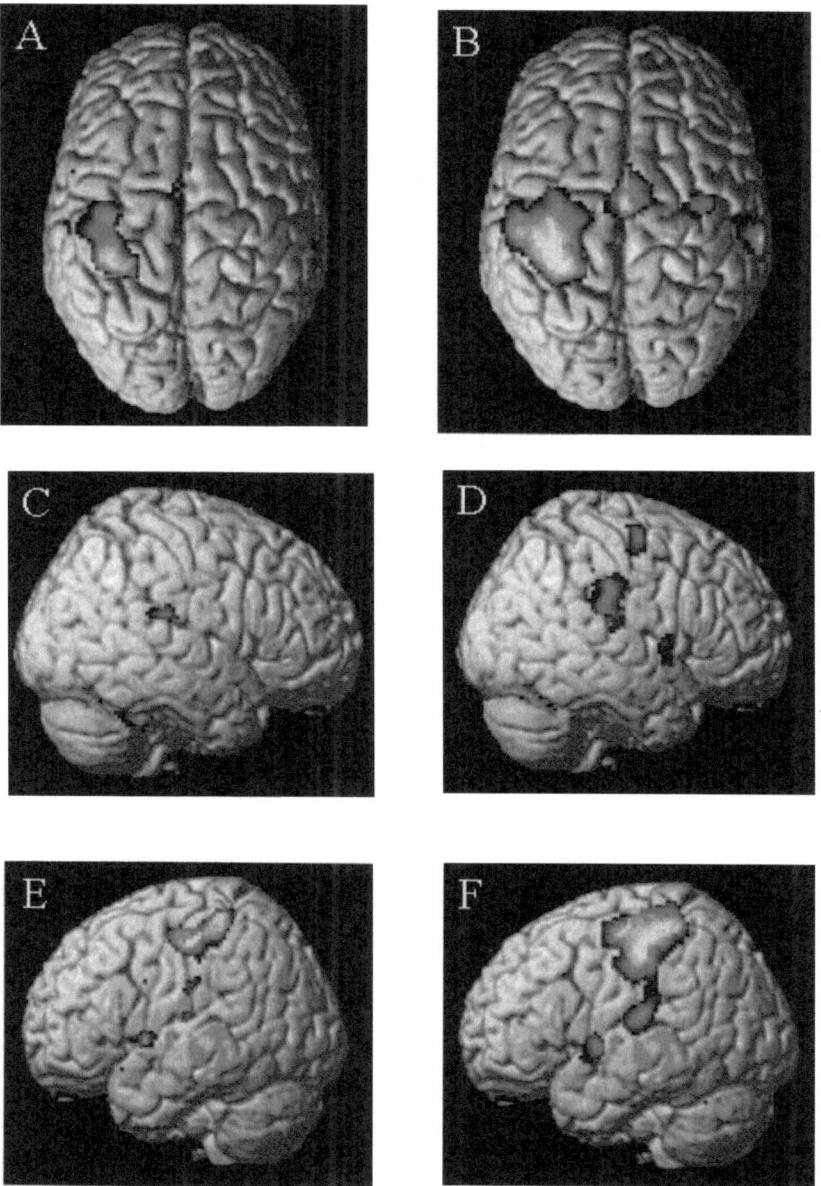

Fig. 6. Brain patterns of cortical activations on a rendered brain in right-handed healthy volunteers (**A, C, E**) and in right-handed PPMS patients (**B, D, F**) during the performance of a simple motor task with their clinically unimpaired right hand. In both groups, a widespread activation of several areas of the sensorimotor network (including the contralateral primary and secondary sensorimotor cortex and the supplementary motor area) is visible. In MS patients, larger activations of these areas and recruitment of additional regions (such as the ipsilateral middle frontal gyrus) are evident

in patients with PPMS after tissue injury, the extent of such changes should be greater with increasing volumes of T2-visible lesions and severity of intrinsic tissue damage of brain T2-visible lesions, brain NABT and cervical cord damage. Consistently with this hypothesis, we found strong correlations between the extent of the fMRI activations of several sensorimotor areas and several MR metrics of structural damage of the brain and the cervical cord. These findings suggest that not only brain, but also cord pathology can induce cortical changes with the potential to limit the functional impact of the disease.

Conclusions

FMRI has the potential to provide important information about cortical reorganization following MS tissue damage which should improve our understanding of the factors associated with the progressive accumulation of irreversible disability in MS. Although the role of cortical reorganization in limiting the functional impact of structural damage in MS is still not definitively proven, the available data support the concept that cortical adaptive responses may have an important role in compensating for tissue damage in MS. They also suggest that the rate of accumulation of disability in MS may be a function not only of tissue loss, but also of progressive failure of the adaptive capacity of the cortex. In particular, the lack or progressive exhaustion of the "classical" adaptive mechanisms and the need of "second order" compensatory areas may be among the factors contributing to the accumulation of irreversible clinical deficits.

References

1. Arnold DL, Matthews PM, Francis G, Antel J (1990) Proton magnetic resonance spectroscopy of human brain in vivo in the evaluation of multiple sclerosis: assessment of the load of disease. Magn Reson Med 14:154-159
2. De Stefano N, Narayanan S, Francis GS et al (2001) Evidence of axonal damage in the early stages of multiple sclerosis and its relevance to disability. Arch Neurol 58:65-70
3. Filippi M, Bozzali M, Gambini A et al (2002) Whole brain N-acetylaspartate concentrations are reduced in patients presenting with clinically isolated syndromes suggestive of MS. J Neurol 249(Suppl 1):I/209
4. Ferguson B, Matyszak MK, Esiri MM, Perry VH (1997) Axonal damage in acute multiple sclerosis lesions. Brain 120:393-399
5. Trapp BD, Ransohoff R, Rudick R (1999) Axonal pathology in multiple sclerosis: relationship to neurologic disability. Curr Opin Neurol 12:295-302
6. Kidd D, Barkhof F, McConnel R et al (1999) Cortical lesions in multiple sclerosis. Brain 122:17-26
7. Brownell B, Hughes JT (1962) The distribution of plaques in the cerebrum in multiple sclerosis. J Neurol Neurosurg Psychiatry 25:315-320
8. Peterson JW, Bo L, Mork S et al (2001) Transected neurites, apoptotic neurons, and reduced inflammation in cortical multiple sclerosis lesions. Ann Neurol 50:389-400
9. Ge Y, Grossman RI, Udupa JK et al (2002) Magnetization transfer ratio histogram analysis of normal-appearing gray matter and normal-appearing white matter in multiple sclerosis. J Comput Assist Tomogr 26:62-68

10. Cercignani M, Bozzali M, Iannucci G et al (2001) Magnetisation transfer ratio and mean diffusivity of normal appearing white and grey matter from patients with multiple sclerosis. J Neurol Neurosurg Psychiatry 70:311-317

11. Bozzali M, Cercignani M, Sormani MP et al (2002) Quantification of brain gray matter damage in different MS phenotypes by use of diffusion tensor MR imaging. AJNR Am J Neuroradiol 23:985-988

12. Sarchielli P, Presciutti O, Tarducci R et al (2002) Localized (1)H magnetic resonance spectroscopy in mainly cortical gray matter of patients with multiple sclerosis. J Neurol 249:902-910

13. Lassmann H, Brück W, Lucchinetti C, Rodriguez M (1997) Remyelination in multiple sclerosis. Mult Scler 3:133-136

14. Waxman SG, Ritchie JM (1993) Molecular dissection of the myelinated axon. Ann Neurol 33:121-136

15. De Stefano N, Narayanan S, Matthews PM et al (1999) In vivo evidence for axonal dysfunction remote from focal cerebral demyelination of the type seen in multiple sclerosis. Brain 122:1933-1939

16. Waxman SG (2001) Acquired channelopathies in nerve injury and MS. Neurology 56:1621-1627

17. Ogawa S, Menon RS, Tank DW et al (1993) Functional brain mapping by blood oxygenation level-dependent contrast magnetic resonance imaging. A comparison of signal characteristics with a biophysical model. Biophys J 64:803-812

18. Ogawa S, Menon RS, Kim SG, Ugurbil K (1998) On the characteristics of functional magnetic resonance imaging of the brain. Annu Rev Biophys Biomol Struct 27:447-474

19. Filippi M, Rocca MA (2002) Functional magnetic resonance imaging. In: Filippi M, Comi G (eds) Primary progressive multiple sclerosis. Springer, Milan, pp 111-124

20. Vanzetta I, Grinvald A (1999) Increased cortical oxidative metabolism due to sensory stimulation: implications for functional brain imaging. Science 286:1555-1558

21. Bandettini PA, Jesmanowicz A, Wong EC, Hyde JS (1993) Processing strategies for time-course data sets in functional MRI of the human brain. Magn Reson Med 30:161-173

22. Worsley KJ, Friston KJ (1995) Analysis of fMRI time-series revisited-again. Neuroimage 2:173-181

23. Filippi M, Paty DW, Kappos L et al (1995) Correlations between changes in disability and T2-weighted brain MRI activity in multiple sclerosis: a follow-up study. Neurology 45:255-260

24. Lycklama à Nijeholt GJ, van Walderveen MA, Castelijns JA et al (1998) Brain and spinal cord abnormalities in multiple sclerosis. Correlation between MRI parameters, clinical subtypes and symptoms. Brain 121:687-697

25. Kappos L, Moeri D, Radue EW et al (1999) Predictive value of gadolinium-enhanced magnetic resonance imaging for relapse rate and changes in disability or impairment in multiple sclerosis: a meta-analysis. Gadolinium MRI Meta-analysis Group. Lancet 353:964-969

26. De Stefano N, Matthews PM, Fu L et al (1998) Axonal damage correlates with disability in patients with relapsing-remitting multiple sclerosis. Results of a longitudinal magnetic resonance spectroscopy study. Brain 121:1469-1477

27. Filippi M (2001) Linking structural, metabolic and functional changes in multiple sclerosis. Eur J Neurol 8:291-297

28. Mainero C, De Stefano N, Iannucci G et al (2001) Correlates of MS disability assessed in vivo using aggregates of MR quantities. Neurology 56:1331-1334

29. Clanet M, Berry I, Boulanouar K (1997) Functional imaging in multiple sclerosis. Int MS J 4:26-32

30. Lee M, Reddy H, Johansen-Berg H et al (2000) The motor cortex shows adaptive functional changes to brain injury from multiple sclerosis. Ann Neurol 47:606-613

31. Noseworthy JH, Lucchinetti C, Rodriguez M, Weinshenker BG (2000) Multiple sclerosis. N Engl J Med 343:938-952

32. Iannucci G, Tortorella C, Rovaris M et al (2000) Prognostic value of MR and magnetization transfer imaging findings in patients with clinically isolated syndromes suggestive of multiple sclerosis at presentation. AJNR Am J Neuroradiol 21:1034-1038

33. Brex PA, Jenkins R, Fox NC et al (2000) Detection of ventricular enlargement in patients at the earliest clinical stage of MS. Neurology 54:1689-1691

34. Filippi M, Inglese M, Rovaris M et al (2000) Magnetization transfer imaging to monitor the evolution of MS: a 1-year follow-up study. Neurology 55:940-946

35. Rudick RA, Fisher E, Lee JC et al (1999) Use of the brain parenchymal fraction to measure whole brain atrophy in relapsing-remitting MS. Multi Scler Collaborative Research Group. Neurology 53:1698-1704

36. Chard DT, Griffin CM, Parker GJ et al (2002) Brain atrophy in clinically early relapsing-remitting multiple sclerosis. Brain 125:327-337

37. Kapeller P, McLean MA, Griffin CM et al (2001) Preliminary evidence for neuronal damage in cortical grey matter and normal appearing white matter in short duration relapsing-remitting multiple sclerosis: a quantitative MR spectroscopic imaging study. J Neurol 248:131-138

38. Werring DJ, Bullmore ET, Toosy AT et al (2000) Recovery from optic neuritis is associated with a change in the distribution of cerebral response to visual stimulation: a functional magnetic resonance imaging study. J Neurol Neurosurg Psychiatry 68:441-449

39. Filippi M, Rocca MA, Falini A et al (2002) A functional MRI study of patients at presentation with clinically isolated syndromes suggestive of multiple sclerosis. J Neurol 249 (Suppl 1):I/20

40. Pantano P, Iannetti GD, Caramia F et al (2002) Cortical motor reorganization after a single clinical attack of multiple sclerosis. Brain 125:1607-1615

41. Mesulam MM (1998) From sensation to cognition. Brain 121:1013-1052

42. McDonald WI, Compston A, Edan G et al (2001) Recommended diagnostic criteria for multiple sclerosis: guidelines from the International Panel on the Diagnosis of Multiple Sclerosis. Ann Neurol 50:121-127

43. Reddy H, Narayanan S, Matthews PM et al (2000) Relating axonal injury to functional recovery in MS. Neurology 54:236-239

44. Filippi M, Iannucci G, Tortorella C et al (1999) Comparison of MS clinical phenotypes using conventional and magnetization transfer MRI. Neurology 52:588-594

45. Rocca MA, Falini A, Colombo B et al (2002) Adaptive functional changes in the cerebral cortex of patients with nondisabling multiple sclerosis correlate with the extent of brain structural damage. Ann Neurol 51:330-339

46. Filippi M, Rocca MA, Colombo B et al (2002) Functional magnetic resonance imaging correlates of fatigue in multiple sclerosis. Neuroimage 15:559-567

47. Rombouts SA, Lazeron RH, Scheltens P et al (1998) Visual activation patterns in patients with optic neuritis: an fMRI pilot study. Neurology 50:1896-1899

48. Langkilde AR, Frederiksen JL, Rostrup E, Larsson HB (2002) Functional MRI of the visual cortex and visual testing in patients with previous optic neuritis. Eur J Neurol 9:277-286

49. Reddy H, Narayanan S, Arnoutelis R et al (2000) Evidence for adaptive functional changes in the cerebral cortex with axonal injury from multiple sclerosis. Brain 123:2314-2320

50. Filippi M, Rocca MA, Minicucci L et al (1999) Magnetization transfer imaging of patients with definite MS and negative conventional MRI. Neurology 52:845-848

51. Filippi M, Rocca MA, Pagani E et al (2002) Functional cortical changes in patients with MS and non-specific findings on conventional MRI scans of the brain. Neuroimage, in press

52. Liepert J, Dettmers C, Terborg C, Weiller C (2001) Inhibition of ipsilateral motor cortex during phasic generation of low force. Clin Neurophysiol 112:114-121

53. Lowe MJ, Phillips MD, Lurito JT et al (2002) Multiple sclerosis: low-frequency temporal blood oxygen level-dependent fluctuations indicate reduced functional connectivity initial results. Radiology 224:184-192

54. Reddy H, Narayanan S, Mitsumori T et al (2002) Functional brain reorganization for hand movement in patients with multiple sclerosis: defining distinct effects of injury and disability. Brain, in press

55. Staffen W, Mair A, Zauner H et al (2002) Cognitive function and fMRI in patients with multiple sclerosis: evidence for compensatory cortical activation during an attention task. Brain 125:1275-1282

59. Thompson AJ, Montalban X, Barkhof F et al (2000) Diagnostic criteria for primary progressive multiple sclerosis: a position paper. Ann Neurol 47:831-835

57. Thompson AJ, Kermode AG, Wicks D et al (1991) Major differences in the dynamics of primary and secondary progressive multiple sclerosis. Ann Neurol 29:53-62

58. Kidd D, Thorpe JW, Kendall BE et al (1996) MRI dynamics of brain and spinal cord in progressive multiple sclerosis. J Neurol Neurosurg Psychiatry 60:15-19

59. Stevenson VL, Miller DH, Rovaris M et al (1999) Primary and transitional progressive MS: a clinical and MRI cross-sectional study. Neurology 52:839-845

60. Stevenson VL, Miller DH, Leary SM et al (2000) One year follow up study of primary and transitional progressive multiple sclerosis. J Neurol Neurosurg Psychiatry 68:713-718

61. Leary SM, Davie CA, Parker GJ et al (1999) ^{1}H magnetic resonance spectroscopy of normal appearing white matter in primary progressive multiple sclerosis. J Neurol 246:1023-1026

62. Leary SM, Silver NC, Stevenson VL et al (1999) Magnetisation transfer of normal appearing white matter in primary progressive multiple sclerosis. Mult Scler 5:313-316

63. Rovaris M, Bozzali M, Santuccio G et al (2001) In vivo assessment of the brain and cervical cord pathology of patients with primary progressive multiple sclerosis. Brain 124:2540-2549

64. Rocca MA, Matthews PM, Caputo D et al (2002) Evidence for widespread movement-associated functional MRI changes in patients with PPMS. Neurology 58:866-872

65. Filippi M, Rocca MA, Falini A et al (2002) Correlations between structural CNS damage and functional MRI changes in primary progressive MS. Neuroimage 15:537-546

66. Rao SM, Binder JR, Bandettini PA et al (1993) Functional magnetic resonance imaging of complex human movements. Neurology 43:2311-2318

67. Paus T, Petrides M, Evans AC, Meyer E (1993) Role of the human anterior cingulate cortex in the control of oculomotor, manual, and speech responses: a positron emission tomography study. J Neurophysiol 70:453-469

68. Jenkins IH, Brooks DJ, Nixon PD et al (1994) Motor sequence learning: a study with positron emission tomography. J Neurosci 14:3775-3790

69. de Gelder B (2000) Neuroscience. More to seeing than meets the eye. Science 289:1148-1149

70. van Waesberghe JH, Kamphorst W, De Groot CJ et al (1999) Axonal loss in multiple sclerosis lesions: magnetic resonance imaging insights into substrates of disability. Ann Neurol 46:747-754

71. Pierpaoli C, Jezzard P, Basser PJ et al (1996) Diffusion tensor MR imaging of the human brain. Radiology 201:637-648

Chapter 7

In vivo Microscopic Imaging of Multiple Sclerosis with High Field MRI

A. Kangarlu, K.W. Rammohan, E.C. Bourekas, D.W. Chakeres

Introduction

Acquiring the ability to visualize areas of demyelination in the brains of patients with multiple sclerosis (MS) by magnetic resonance imaging (MRI) marked a turning point in the diagnosis of this disease. MRI has enabled the systematic examination of distribution and time-dependent characteristics that lead to the development of long-term clinical disability in MS patients. An understanding of this series of events permits a qualitative and quantitative evaluation by MRI of the effects of therapeutic strategies [1]. Many of the early MRI studies examined the sensitivity of the MRI technique in detecting lesions of MS [2] only. The long-term natural history of MS has also been studied by MRI. It has long been evident that relapses of MS as evident on MRI occur regularly, but that only a small fraction of such exacerbations manifest clinically. Therefore, MRI is essential to directly monitor the progression of disease. Drugs under investigation for their efficacy have been examined for their ability to modify the MRI profile [3], and a favorable effect visible on MRI has become an expected effect of such drugs. However, a disparity has been identified in numerous studies and over the last decade: it has become increasingly evident that lesions seen on conventional MRI may correlate poorly with clinical disability. Therefore, there remain significant imaging challenges to better characterize MS patients by MRI. Defining the white matter lesions is not the complete story.

Nevertheless, other techniques of MRI have been found to be essential in patient management and therapy studies in demyelinating disorders, and for a similar reason: that many imaging findings occur without associated clinical symptoms [4, 5]. MR imaging thus allows a more objective assessment of the activity of the disease. Among the imaging techniques developed to date, high-field (HF) MRI is recognized as the one with the highest potential to offer specificity in the correlation between detected plaques and clinical disabilities. The traditional high field that extended up to 4 T has now been substantially increased to 7 and 8 T for human application [6].

The safe exposure of more than 500 human subjects to these field strengths allows the potentials of HF MRI for MS diagnosis and treatment to be explored [7, 8]. In spite of the fact that a number of technological challenges such as high susceptibility, RF coil, mode inhomogeneity, and higher specific absorption rates (SAR) will require more work in order to make this field strength diagnostically viable, the advantages of HF MRI must be fully scrutinized for human MS studies [9].

The value of HF MRI has also been demonstrated in imaging work at 9.4 T on experimental allergic encephalomyelitis (EAE), the animal model for investigation on the pathology of MS [10]. The perivascular cuffs of inflammation and demyelination visualized in this work indicate the potential of this technique in visualizing microscopic pathology in MS. In addition, MRI provides the opportunity to evaluate normal-appearing white matter (NAWM) that may actually be pathologic when assessed using more quantitative methods. The capability to evaluate the NAWM has been limited at fields up to 1.5 T. This being so, our intention is ultimately to evaluate HF MRI for promising measures such as diffusion coefficients, magnetization ratios, and T2 relaxation times for their potential to quantify the microscopic disease within NAWM. This may help document disease activity within NAWM that may correlate better with the clinical disease status. MRI at 4 T has already been performed on MS patients [11] and given some indication of the unique information attainable at high field strength. Our long-term goal is to develop all the capabilities of HF MRI for detection, distinction, and evaluation of MS and ultimately promote MRI as a tool to distinguish various types of clinical disease with better correlation between imaging and clinical disability. To date, we have completed the evaluation of 8-T MRI as a tool for MS patient imaging and have found areas of strength in which unique findings are made in plaque visualization.

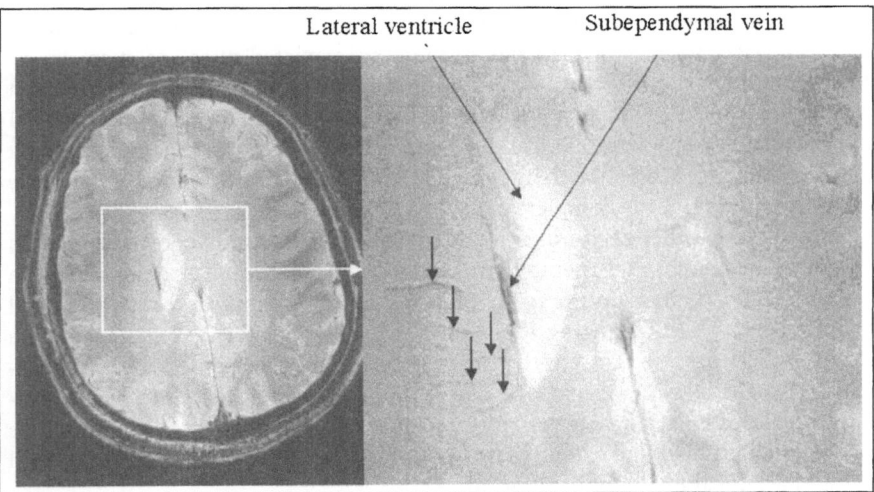

Fig. 1. Normal 8-T GE axial MRI. The image to the *left* is a 1024 × 1024 axial GE 8-T MR image centered at the level of the upper lateral ventricles. The *right* image is the magnified region outlined in the *white box* on the left image. Many small, linear low-signal regions (*short black arrows*) are seen, representing the medullary veins of the corona radiata. They radiate towards the subependymal veins at the margin of the lateral ventricle. Routinely, hundreds of these vessels are visible. There are no white matter lesions in this image

Materials and Methods

A 16-strut RF coil of transverse electromagnetic (TEM) design was used for these studies. A group of six patients with known MS were selected within the context of an Investigational Review Board protocol. All patients signed informed consent. The imaging was performed using the TEM coil for excitation and acquisition of the images with an 8-T/80-cm whole-body MRI scanner. The TEM coil was utilized in either two- or four-port excitation/receive mode. Typical gradient echo (GE) image acquisition parameters at 8 T were TR = 750 ms, TE = 12 ms, FOV = 512 × 512 and 1024 × 1024 matrix, receiver bandwidth = 50 kHz, single excitation, no averaging, slice thickness = 2 mm, flip angle = 20 °. The fast spin echo equivalent, the so-called rapid acquisition by relaxation enhancement or RARE sequence, was used to acquire images with typical parameters of TR = 500 ms, TE = 22 ms, FOV = 512 × 512, receiver bandwidth = 70 KHz, single excitation, echo train length = 4, slice thickness = 2 mm. A number of 1.5-T images of some of the patients were available for comparison with the 8-T results. In evaluation of the 8-T images, a number of distinct features of HF MRI such as lesion appearance, size, and distribution, appearance and relationship of the deep medullary veins, and their distribution to the lesion were considered.

Results and Discussion

A large number of normal volunteers have been imaged with the 8-T/80-cm whole-body scanner since 1998. In the process of imaging normal volunteers and patients with MS we noted that there was prominent visualization of vascular structures representing medullary veins and subependymal veins (Fig. 1). This imaging work was performed in order to establish both the safety and human imaging protocols at this field strength.

For the MS patients, the areas of white matter demyelination were seen as high-signal-intensity regions on both the GE and RARE images (Figs. 2 and 3). The plaques were identified in typical locations for demyelinating lesions, including the corpus callosum and the periventricular region. We did not evaluate the posterior fossa structures in detail, partly due to coil limitations in evaluating that region. The distribution of the lesions seen on lower-field MR images was similar to that in the high-field studies, but we did not have comparisons for all of the patients. The MS changes were high in signal intensity on both the GE and the RARE sequences. There was a clear relationship between the demyelinating lesions and the deep venous system. The medullary veins were seen as low-signal-intensity, branching linear structures radiating from the subependymal veins toward the gray-white matter interface more peripherally. Central veins were seen as low-signal-intensity linear structures in the mid portions of the plaques. The high-signal regions paralleled the veins radiating from the margins of the lateral ventricles.

The search for abnormalities in NAWM is a new focus of research. Important

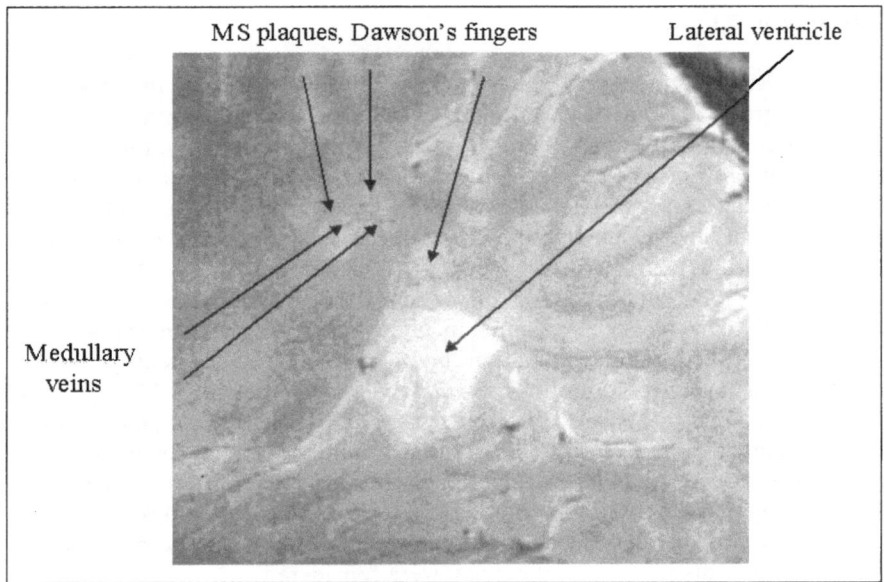

Fig. 2. Sagittal 8-T GE MRI of Dawson's fingers. This is a sagittal 512 × 512 GE image centered on the trigone of the lateral ventricle. The cerebral spinal fluid spaces demonstrate the highest signal intensity, followed by the gray matter and then the white matter. Regions of increased signal intensity forming Dawson's finger MS plaques are visible in the periventricular region and extending along the medullary veins. The veins are seen as small low-signal foci centered in the plaques

insights may be obtained by scrutinizing visible white matter lesions in greater detail as well. HF MRI with its high-resolution in vivo capability has provided a new opportunity for such scrutiny. It is well known that through a series of immune responses, allergens in the blood stimulate mast cells and basophils to secrete various chemicals and hormones such as histamine, leukotrienes, and tumor necrosis factor. It is also known that the chemicals secreted by the activated basophils and mast cells can cause a significant increase in the permeability of capillaries. It would be valuable to establish whether compromise in the permeability of the blood-brain barrier (BBB) occurs at the level of venous structures and whether it is detectable by HF MRI. Elucidation of such an occurrence could help determine specifically the elements participating in the regulation of blood-brain permeability. Thus, animal models could be developed to study increased permeabilities in the BBB. The observation of BBB breakdown would provide direct evidence of the disease etiology. This capability would enable us to address the role of the activated mast cells in demyelination. The natural continuation of this work would also allow quantification of the role of the mediators (histamine and protease) in MS and answer the question of whether an external factor triggers the release from the perivascular mast cells of these potential mediators.

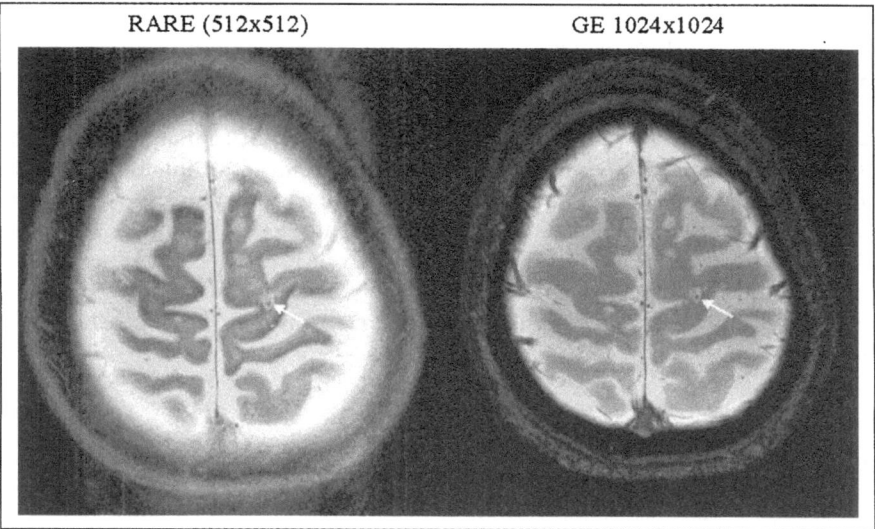

Fig. 3. Comparison of the RARE and GE axial 8-T images. The *left* figure is a RARE 512 × 512 matrix image. The *right* figure is a 1024 × 1024 GE image at the same level. Multiple MS plaques (*white arrow*) are visible as high signal regions with small, low-signal-intensity veins centrally. The gray-white matter differentiation is better on the RARE images than on the GE images. The gray matter is lower in signal intensity than the white matter. Both demonstrate similar signal patterns related to the plaque changes. Note that a central vein is seen in nearly every high-signal-intensity lesion

From pathologic studies, the distribution of MS plaques has been known for years to parallel the venous structures. This phenomenon has been called "Dawson's fingers." Recently, this distribution has been described using magnetic susceptibility contrast-enhanced MR imaging [5, 12]. Our technique produces similar images, but without the more complicated magnetic susceptibility-based imaging techniques. The HF GE images are highly sensitive to the deoxyhemo-globin of the venous structures. The deoxyhemoglobin is paramagnetic and leads to local field inhomogeneities and secondary loss of signal intensity due to T2* spin dephasing. The linking of the lesion and the vessel pattern distribution may help differentiate small regions of demyelination from infarction, since the lesions associated particularly with arterial disease do not localize on the medullary venous system. This study demonstrates that 8-T imaging can generate high-quality images of demyelination.

Conclusions

High-resolution HF MRI has demonstrated the characteristic relationship between the lesions and the deep venous system. The plaques are centered around microvessels, and this could help identify the etiology of this white matter disease. The perivenular nature of the MS plaque was defined ante mortem in patients using HFMRI, something that until now was possible only by pathologic examination of the plaque. This permitted MS lesions to be distinguished from small-vessel-disease-related lesions of the deep white matter (lacunar infarcts and leukoaraiosis). This also permits the classification of MS according to pathologic subtype, since a central vein as a feature of the plaque is only observed in types I and II according to recent classifications of the pathology of multiple sclerosis [13]. These preliminary studies show a promising role for HF MRI in better defining the plaque architecture and pathology, enabling better selection of patients for clinical trials, and following the effects of treatment on the clinical course of the disease.

References

1. McFarland HF, Stone LA, Calabresi PA et al (1996) MRI studies of multiple sclerosis: implications for the natural history of the disease and for monitoring effectiveness of experimental therapies. Mult Scler 2:198-205
2. Frank JA, Bash C, Stone L et al (1996) Evaluation of magnetic resonance imaging sensitivity in patients with relapsing remitting multiple sclerosis: baseline versus Betaseron treatment trials. Acad Radiol 3S:S173-175
3. Richert ND, Zierak MC, Bash CN et al (2000) MRI and clinical activity in MS patients after terminating treatment with interferon beta-1b. Mult Scler 6:86-90
4. Filippi M, Tortorella C, Rovaris M et al (2000) Changes in the normal appearing brain tissue and cognitive impairment in multiple sclerosis. J Neurol Neurosurg Psychiatry. 68:157-161
5. Tan IL, van Schijndel RA, Pouwels PJ et al (2000) AJNR Am J Neuroradiol 21:1039-1042
6. Robitaille P-ML, Abduljalil AM, Kangarlu A et al (1998) Human magnetic resonance Imaging at 8T. NMR Biomed 11:263-265
7. Kangarlu A, Robitaille PML (2000) MR venography in multiple sclerosis. Biological effects and health implications in magnetic resonance imaging. Concepts Magn Reson 12:321-359
8. Kangarlu A, Burgess RE, Zhu H et al (1999) Cognitive, cardiac and physiological safety studies in ultra high field magnetic resonance imaging. J Magn Reson Imag 17:1407-1416
9. Kangarlu A, Baertlein BA, Lee R et al (1999) Dielectric resonance phenomena in ultra high field magnetic resonance imaging. J Comp Assist Tomogr 23:820-831
10. Gareau PJ, Wymore AC, Cofer GP, Johnson GA (2002) Imaging inflammation: direct visualization of perivascular cuffing in EAE by magnetic resonance microscopy. J Magn Reson Imaging 16:28-36
11. Pan JW, Coyle PK, Bashir K et al (2002) Metabolic differences between multiple sclerosis subtypes measured by quantitative MR spectroscopy. Mult Scler 8:200-206
12. Reichenbach JR, Barth M, Haacke EM et al (2000) High-resolution MR venography at 3.0 Tesla. J Comput Assist Tomogr 24:949-957
13. Lucchinetti C, Brück W, Parisi J et al (2000) Heterogeneity of multiple sclerosis lesions: implications for the pathogenesis of demyelination. Ann Neurol 47:707-17

Subject Index